HEART-ACHES

Heart Disease and the
Psychology of the Broken
Heart

HEART-ACHES

Heart Disease and the
Psychology of the Broken
Heart

RUEDIGER DAHLKE, M.D.
Translated by Petra Michel

SENTIENT PUBLICATIONS

First Sentient Publications edition 2025

Copyright © 1996 by Ruediger Dahlke

All rights reserved. This book, or parts thereof, may not be reproduced in any form without permission, except in the case of brief quotations embodied in critical articles and reviews.

A paperback original

Book design by Laura Waltje
Cover Design by Laura Waltje
Cover Illustration by Jorm Sangsorn

Library of Congress Control Number: 2024948528
Publisher's Cataloging-in-Publication Data
Names: Dahlke, Ruediger, author. | Michel, Petra, translator.

Title: Heart-aches : heart disease and the psychology of the broken heart / Ruediger Dahlke, MD; translated by Petra Michel.

Description: Includes bibliographical references and index. | Boulder, CO: Sentient Publications, 2025.

Identifiers: LCCN: 2024948656 | ISBN: 978-1-59181-342-2 (print) | 978-1-59181-343-9 (epub)
Subjects: LCSH Heart--Diseases--Prevention. | Heart--Diseases--Popular works. | Heart--Diseases--Psychosomatic aspects. | Holistic medicine. | Mind and body. | Psychophysiology. | BISAC HEALTH & FITNESS / Diseases & Conditions / Heart | MEDICAL / Holistic Medicine | BODY, MIND & SPIRIT / Healing / General | SELF-HELP / Self-Management / Stress Management | PHILOSOPHY / Mind & Body
Classification: LCC RA776 .D3415 2025 | DDC 613/.0434--dc23

SENTIENT PUBLICATIONS
A Limited Liability Company
PO Box 1851
Boulder, CO 80306
www.sentientpublications.com

*I would like to thank Dr. Robert Hössl, M.D. and my wife Margit for their support and contributions to this book.
In addition, I would like to thank Ms. Alexandra Steinbeis, Dr Isolde Burgey, M.D., my sister Angela Stargalla, and my father, as well as my patients for the many suggestions and inspiration that formed the basis for this work.*

Contents

Part 1 — 1
1. Solve et Coagula — 3
2. The Disease of the Century — 5
3. The Cultural and Medical History — 14
4. Symptoms as an Expression of Inner Reality — 22
   - 4.1 Evaluation of Symptoms — 22
   - 4.2 Symptoms as Companions on the Path — 24
   - 4.3 "Causes" of Symptoms — 26
   - 4.4 Medical Principle of the Conservation of Energy and Its Shadow — 28
   - 4.5 Form and Meaning — 33
   - 4.6 The Daily Pact with the Devil — 34
   - 4.7 Symptoms—A Summary — 36
5. The Language of the Heart in the Bible — 38
6. The Heart in Timeless Words — 42
7. The Heart and Love — 54

Part 2 — 68
I. The Language of the Heart — 69
1. The Heart's Structure and How It Works — 70
2. The Heart Out of Balance — 81
3. Constrictions of the Heart — 86
   - 3.1 Angina Pectoris—The Narrow Heart — 86
   - 3.2 Heart Attack—The Breaking Heart — 97
   - 3.3 Therapy for the Heart Attack — 111
4. The Embattled Heart — 120
   - 4.1 Rheumatic Carditis and Other Forms of Heart Inflammation — 122
   - 4.2 The Weapons of Orthodox Medicine — 132
5. The Defective Heart — 139
   - 5.1. Congenital Heart Defects and Responsibility — 139
   - 5.2 Various Congenital Heart Defects — 141
     - 5.2.1 Defects of the Heart Septum — 141
     - 5.2.2 Problems with Old Paths — 146
     - 5.2.3 Alarming Reminders of Old Times — 147
   - 5.3 Constrictions and Leaking Spots — 150
     - 5.3.1 Stenoses or Bottlenecks — 151
     - 5 3.2 Regurgitations or Leaking Valves — 161
6. The Heart Out of Rhythm — 169
   - 6.1 Problems at the Top of the Hierarchy — 175
   - 6.2 Competition of the Hierarchy — 178
   - 6.3 Paroxysmal Tachycardia—Racing Attacks of the Heart — 180
   - 6.4 Extrasystoles—Stumbling Blocks on the Path of the Heart — 182
   - 6.5 Flutter and Fibrillation — 184
   - 6.6 Mechanical Block Busters — 188
7. Cardiac Insufficiency—The Failing Heart — 194
8. Further Problems That Touch the Heart — 202
   - 8.1 Degeneration of the Heart — 202
   - 8.2 Fatty Degeneration of the Heart — 203
   - 8.3 Wind That Goes to the Heart — 205
9. Cardiac Neurosis—Fear of the Heart — 208

10. Closing Observations on Heart Problems	220
II. The Organic Language of the Circulatory System	223
1. Structure and Control	224
2. The Basic Structure of Blood Pressure	229
2.1 The Blood—Symbol of Life	229
2.2 Vessel Walls—Symbols of Limitation and Resistance	231
3. Hypotension—Life Without Tension	233
4. Weakness of the Connective Tissue Varicose Veins—Thrombosis	241
5. Therapies for Low Pressure and Connective Tissue	248
6. Hypertension—Life Under Pressure	256
6.1 Figures and Symptoms	256
6.2 External and Internal Pressure	263
6.3 Hypertension and Communication—The Language of the Heart	266
6.4 The Redemption of Pressure—A Chance for Development	273
7. High and Low Pressure—Hand in Hand	279
8. Further Problems in the Course of the Circle	283
Part 3	286
I. Cardiovascular Therapies	287
1. Fundamental Considerations of Medication	288
2. Diet	292
3. Fasting as Therapy and Path	294
4. Inner and Outer Movement	297
5. Spiritual-Emotional Exercises on the Path to the Healed Heart	299
II. The Path of the Heart	303
1. Love	304
Endnotes	309
Bibliography	312
Index	314

Part 1

1.
Solve et Coagula

Our culture views heart trouble as a physical metaphor for heartache; this truism of folk wisdom finds its expression in poetry, proverbs, and everyday conversation. However, it is also an unproven scientific statement from the perspective of modem medicine. This book addresses the tension between the self-evident everyday experience of common feeling and the rigorous proof required by university medicine.

In the process, we can profit from both perspectives if we accept from the very outset that both sides make valuable contributions to our better understanding. However, the foundations of these contributions are completely different. The sole basis for our common feeling and for folk medicine is almost always personal experience, an experience which suggests that the pangs of love manifest themselves specifically in the heart and not in some other organ (such as the liver or the brain). In contrast, scientific medicine relies almost entirely on empirical observation and measurement, and so finds it difficult to integrate a phenomenon such as love at all. Rather, scientific medicine can impart much valuable information about the structure and manner in which the heart functions. As we investigate the more subtle aspects of cardiovascular problems, we should try to consider both of these perspectives simultaneously (although it might not be possible to reconcile them) in order to paint a comprehensive picture of the heart, its themes, and its problems.

Heart-Aches

In accordance with the ancient wisdom of alchemy *solve et coagula* (dissolve and bind), we will use the analytic approach of science to investigate the problem's various parts. After this step of dissolution (the analysis), the images from folk medicine and mythology will help us to reassemble the individual stones in the mosaic, building a complete picture. It is only this synthesis that imparts real value to the analysis and demonstrates that the whole is much more than the sum of it's parts. It seems that human life is far more than a collection of physio-chemical processes—just as the heart is more than a mere collection of muscles. The danger of orthodox medicine is that it only uses physio-chemical measurements and interpretation, while the weakness of alternative therapies is to disregard them entirely.

Now seems to be the right time for a step towards the integration of these two perspectives. In view of a significant increase in the number of symptoms that seem to be linked directly to emotional factors, orthodox medicine has made a focused attempt to get a grip on the psychological dimension of disease. On the other hand, there is a strong and expanding movement in the general population towards folk medicine. Through this movement, people are finding their way towards spirituality, which views everything in its spiritual-emotional dimension.

The original meaning of the word *symptom* derives from the Greek *sympfoma*—coming *together,* the coincidence, or circumstance of an illness—and it also suggests such an activity. A symptom is the visible and tangible manifestation of an illness, where all of the underlying problems converge and find their symbolic expression (from Greek *symballein,* meaning to throw together). The heart is certainly the most suitable organ to illustrate a synthesis of these perspectives since throughout the ages it has been viewed as the center of the human being, a center in which everything comes *together* and becomes one.

2.

The Disease of the Century

These days, considerable mention is made of the Disease of the Century. Various types of cancer—or most recently, AIDS—are often referred to in this context. There is certainly some truth to such classifications but, if we are honest, this dubious honor should really be bestowed upon the diseases of the heart and circulatory system.

These diseases have been on the increase since the beginning of the twentieth century and continue to grow in importance. Switzerland is representative of industrialized nations: death from arteriosclerosis (the basis of heart attack and many other conditions) tripled there in the years 1901 to 1944; cancer increased by "only" fifty percent; deaths caused by tuberculosis and other infectious diseases even declined by fifty percent. In 1947, some form of heart disease was attributed to be the cause of thirty percent of all fatalities. According to the latest statistics from the past ten years, in the industrialized nations, every other person will probably die of heart and circulatory-related diseases. There were 2,600 heart attacks reported in Germany during 1948; forty years later there were already between 85,000 and 100,000. According to another statistic, in Germany alone, approximately one thousand people die from cardiovascular disease every day.

Heart-Aches

The most devastating medical problems in the United States also originate in the heart. One can attribute more than half of the deaths in the United States to heart disease and, in 1980 alone, more than a million Americans died of arteriosclerosis and high blood pressure. According to estimates by the American Heart Association, forty to sixty million Americans suffer from high blood pressure, making it the most important medical problem in the country.

According to the United Nations' World Health Organization (WHO), in every industrial nation in the world, more than half the citizens over the age of forty five suffer from high blood pressure. Its epithet is the new epidemic—the number one silent killer. The insidious manner in which this killer works must be why so many people underestimate its power. In contrast, disease and mortality statistics speak in clear and direct terms. Employment offices can present stacks of dry figures that prove conclusively that blood-pressure-related problems contribute to disability and incapacity. Therefore, it should also be obvious that corresponding medical costs are also at the head of the list. In 1980, more than eighty billion dollars was spent dealing with heart and circulatory problems in the United States alone.

Although such heartless statistics, filled with lifeless figures, can hardly convey a picture of the real situation, they are recognized as a form of scientific language. They often make more of an impression on people of our time (politicians, for example) than heart-rending stories of suffering and personal tragedy.

Therefore, one should conclude that a particular group of diseases (a group that can develop very rapidly) has apparently found a good breeding ground for itself during this century. At the same time, the breeding ground became worse for tuberculosis and so it subsided. If we take a closer look at the flood of figures, we can learn even more from them. They reveal that heart disease steadily increased during the first half of the twentieth century, and show a landslide acceleration at the beginning of the second half. This must mean that the breeding ground for cardiovascular problems has improved dramatically—precisely in our time. The statistics also illustrate a clear shift away from coronary valvular defects during the first half of the century and towards coronary sclerosis (narrowing of the coronary vessels) during the second half

Perhaps the most astonishing and more revealing result of our situation comes from an apparent secondary aspect of the statistics. If WHO informs us tersely that cardiovascular disease is one of the leading causes of death in all the industrialized nations, then the question arises: What about the situation in non-industrialized countries? In fact, there is an impressive contrast provided by the few cultures that still maintain the native customs and life-styles which keep them close to nature. The contrast remains even if one takes into account the fundamentally different living conditions. Cardiovascular disease plays a secondary role in these situations, and high blood pressure does not exist at all.

The result applies equally to these few surviving native cultures, whether we consider the native tribes in Szechwan (Central China), American Indians of the Amazon jungle, Zulus in rural Africa, the Melanesians in New Guinea, or the aborigines of the Polynesian island world. All these peoples share one common factor—their blood pressure does not increase with age, as it almost always does in modem cultures.

Scientists have attempted to attribute such results (which very clearly speak against our civilization) to a great variety of external phenomena—the most common being the lack of salt in the diets of such ancient cultures. Science tends to discount the fact that these people live completely different life-styles and hold value systems that oppose western culture. In the example of the Polynesians, one can clearly see how such purely physical explanations are questionable; they certainly do not lack salt in the middle of their salty oceanic world. Another argument attempts to find the explanation in differing genotypes and variations in constitution, a conclusion also proven erroneous in the light of further examination. While the blood pressure of African-Americans was already very high at the start of the twentieth century, this phenomenon did not simultaneously manifest itself in the Africans who share their genetic roots. In countries such as Nigeria, there was no such thing as high blood pressure. The circumstances have changed today, with Nigeria sharing the same diseases as other industrialized nations. Blood pressure remains low in rural, traditional tribal regions while it increases in the more urbanized areas.

This tendency also shows up in the Navajo Indians of New Mexico and Arizona. As long as they maintain their traditional way of life on the reservation, their blood pressure is normal—lower than that of both white and black Americans. However, their blood pressure adapts to the environment as soon as they migrate to urban surroundings. This phenomenon also occurs in Eskimos who leave their native homeland in Greenland and move to Denmark.

Time and again, investigations of this type serve to illustrate the same correlation. It is up to us to interpret these observations, and possibly the only conclusion we may draw is that cardiovascular diseases—in particular high blood pressure and coronary sclerosis—need our modern industrial world as a breeding ground. We must seriously ask ourselves whether it is our industriousness (from the Latin *industria*) which brings us to an early grave.

The popular counter-argument is that western life expectancy—despite everything—is still higher than that of the native cultures mentioned above, but this argument also has its limits. There are many reasons for the relatively early deaths in those cultures, all of which have nothing to do with cardiovascular problems. This becomes clear through examinations of older tribal members who—in contrast to their 'highly civilized' contemporaries—are free of symptoms. Besides, from the medical perspective regarding the life expectancy of the cells, there is absolutely no reason why we should not live much longer than we do today. Cardiovascular disease is what hinders us the most from achieving a ripe old age.

The Disease of the Century

The above conclusions may seem exaggerated, or in any case premature. However, they point in a direction that is worth exploring. In order to do justice to a symptom, it is important to explore thoroughly the ground on which it develops. Also, this exploration should not be limited to the external-material world alone, as it is the spiritual-emotional factors in particular that make this rapid growth possible. For cardiovascular diseases, it seems clear that it is the collective life-style in our industrial society that shapes this breeding ground. This in no way means that we should blame society. Rather, this is a comprehensive perspective, as Paracelsus could very well see. He felt convinced that the microcosm (a human being) corresponds to everything in the macrocosm (the world) and vice versa. He insisted that a doctor should draw conclusions about the patient's environment from his symptoms as well as the other way around (drawing conclusions about the patient from the environmental symptoms). In this sense, we should be able to find the same fundamental pattern—we can start with someone suffering from heart disease, or we can start with a society suffering from heart trouble.

This form of analysis will even more certainly lead us to our goal: cardiovascular problems are symptoms of our era—much more profoundly and more comprehensively than all the other symptoms that have taken the blame. The person with heart disease is afflicted in his center and a society with heart trouble is consequently sick at its center as well. However, what is the center of our society? What—in addition to the physical symptoms of high blood pressure—are its main problems on a spiritual- emotional level?

People have often attempted to describe the *Zeitgeist* (spirit of the times) with a diagnosis from the psychopathological field. These attempts have often had their kernel of truth. A narcissistic tendency is certainly the characteristic of modern industrial societies and the era that has produced them. Preoccupation with the self is greater today than at any other time in history. While artists in earlier ages worked anonymously for the glory of God, today they sign every work in their own honor. They prefer to become famous, and most people would like to imitate them. In earlier times, honoring God was the purpose for erecting primarily religious structures such as cathedrals, domes, and temples while today, the main purpose for building factories is to raise the balance of one's own bank account. Society admonishes every individual to be the architect of his own fortune. It is an accepted fact of life that the happiness of other people comes to grief now and then. Falling in love with one's own fortune and one's own success qualifies as narcissism. A more mature form of love is oriented towards the other person and so must necessarily lose out in a narcissistic society. The accusation that our society is primarily narcissistic, therefore, suggests that the society has a problem with love.

On the other hand, fear also deserves top billing as a characteristic representative of our age. The Gestalt therapist Rollo May speaks of the fear-obsessed twentieth century and there are many convincing arguments that support this perspective. Anxiety comes from narrowness (from the Latin *angustus*, meaning narrow), and present-day earth is probably more crowded today than at any other time. With the uninterrupted population explosion, this crowding becomes increasingly more oppressive. Wherever things become constricted, pressure also rises—an observation that applies not only in the classroom or at the market place, but also in every vessel and every blood vessel as well. Although the threat from nature has decreased, the overall threat has increased. It is no longer nature that threatens the human race but rather it is the human being which threatens the human race and nature, ultimately threatening itself. The external threat has turned into an internal threat. More threat creates more pressure and the advancing proximity of increased fear. Angina pectoris (constriction within the chest) has thereby been transmuted from an individual symptom into the symbol of an oppressive situation.

As an example, schizophrenia is already the testimony for our age and there is evidence of an international paranoid persecution complex—from the armament race to disturbed relations between both countries and individuals. Evident is a muddle-headed way of thinking as well as an almost hebephrenic feeling of absolute apathy for our mutual future. A lack of relationship to other people is a common disorder and, since it also strikes the center of every society, it should not be surprising that there is a correlation between heart disease and interpersonal relationships. From this point of view, relationship disorders are obviously an important risk factor in heart problems.

On an individual level, the schizophrenic, the anxiety neurotic, and the narcissist embody characteristics of this society. However, all three are burdens to society. The illness of a society should be helpful to it, just as every symptom is ultimately helpful to a patient when one considers the whole process.

This takes us to the broad field of compulsion. A compulsive individual is the best guarantee for the continued functioning of a modern industrial society. He is obedient and willing to adapt and he maintains both himself and the rules of his environment at all times. Reliability and a love of order and precision have become flesh and blood in his person. His conscientiousness, industriousness, punctuality, and honesty are his guarantee of perfect functioning, virtues which lead to success in our times. Our schools and universities are organized to train students in these virtues and, ideally, to produce such people.

Compulsive subordinates are the dream to the powerful people of this world. Who would not want to be reliable, orderly, honest, clean, precise, and conscientious? Parents desire such children and teachers hope for this type of pupil. Foremen promote such apprentices while most professors also prefer this type of student. Politicians are happiest when they have this type of constituency and companies desire this type both as employee and as consumer. The advertising industry makes this ideal palatable to us. Armed against the world—kept beautifully clean and stylish with tons of laundry detergent, sprays, and deodorants—made fit and willing to perform with the appropriate foods—the perfectly average compulsive-neurotic dashes into the daily struggle for existence. She leaves nothing to coincidence as a matter of principle. Every risk is insured away—including life itself. The course of her life is carefully planned in secure, well-defined paths. Managers of building societies and savings accounts are at her side as our ideal person marches securely along in the success lane. She displays good behavior by following fashion as she participates in all the other what-people-should-and-should-not-do games. At the same time, she must take care that not too many playful factors penetrate her life—they could make things somewhat confusing. Everything is under control—most of all, the future. A person must be willing to really put his shoulder to the wheel in order to achieve so much security. Of course, family planning is required here, too. One aims for the career ladder and the objective is to own a condominium as soon as possible. A person has only to be willing to work a bit harder to achieve all of this.

If—in spite of his status and his many symbols of security—such a person does not find the expected happiness at some point, no one else will notice it anyway. Appearances must seem to be in order, the facade remains intact, everything is under control. Only a psychologist could recognize the anxiety of his own inner (emotional) chaos behind such strict order, the panic of his own fate behind the magic of insurance, the fear of playing freely, or fear of rapture and ecstasy behind an impressive love of order. The compulsive person has little in common with such feelings. Ultimately, there are rules and ordinances for everything and a person simply has to obey them. Then he will find recognition everywhere in our (compulsive) society.

Then, this order of rules, regulations, and mandates replaces the natural order. Far too much is prearranged—from the pill, to the occupation, to the parking spot, to the life partner. At the end of life, nearly everything is planned as well. Despite an apparently flawless democracy, the dictates of behavior lead to a form of inner dictatorship. Even if these dictates leave a glimmer of free space, laws guarantee unshakable stability. With time, this condition penetrates all facets of society and personality. From the firm character to the solidified inner structure, the path leads to the hard core of the rigid personality with a correspondingly hard heart. As Alfred Ziegler expressed it: "In an *anacastic* (compulsive neurotic) world, the heart petrifies step by step." The extreme form of a society, completely rigid in its bureaucratic ordinances, harsh laws, and inexorable rules, is analogous to the state of *rigor mortis,* the stiffness of the physical body that occurs after death.

3.

The Cultural and Medical History of the Heart and the Circulatory System

Of course, it is impossible to date the first historical record of the heart but it probably coincides with the beginning of human history. There is a strong analogy between the life history of an individual human being and the development of one's heart. The heart and its vascular system is one of the first organs to develop within the growing embryo, as it circulates the blood of the unborn from the very beginning.

Our ancestors were certainly capable of differentiating between life and death—even at a time when they still dwelt in caves. Even then, they had to distinguish the so-called life signs, to distinguish a sleeping person from a dead one. For this purpose, breath and its movements were significant—as well as body temperature and the blood supply to the skin. If our ancestors had already located the secret of the breath in the thorax, then the heartbeat certainly must have been conspicuous to them as well—particularly since they could feel it within their own chests after any form of exertion. After millennia of development, medical science has still only been able to find one other easily tested essential life sign—the blood pressure.

Cannibalistic customs and sacrificial ceremonies from early in human history suggest that man already understood the importance of the heart as the source of life. Primitive man ate the hearts of both animals and humans to acquire the courage and strength of their previous owners. The apparent basis for this act was the lore that both of these qualities dwelt in the heart. Long before our time, the Aztecs cut out the hearts of captive warriors and sacrificed them to their god as the most precious part of their spoils.

One of the first references to the significance of the heart lies in the 4,500 year-old epic *Gilgamesh,* wherein the heart is associated with the divine nature of the human being. The ancient writings of the Hindu tradition—probably significantly older—draw an even finer distinction. *The Vedas* purport that the heart chakra—*Anahata,* the middle of the seven energy centers—corresponds to the heavenly city of Brahmaputra. Both spiritual and emotional life pour out of it, as it is the place where one can establish a connection to the divine. The ancient Egyptians considered the heart to be the seat of the conscience and it was for this reason that the goddess Maat weighed it after death. The embalmer cut it out of the body and replaced it with a stone scarab—the symbol of unity and therefore of the Sun God. Some of the noble European families—such as the Hapsburgs—still observe the custom of burying the heart (as the most important organ) separate from the body. The Bavarian Royal House of the Wittelsbachs buries the hearts of deceased family members in the Chapel of the Black Madonna, which stands in their family village Altötting.

The ancient Greeks considered the heart to be the seat of emotion and passion. Plato called it the site of the immortal soul and Aristotle referred to it as the organ of feeling and emotion. Finally, the Bible speaks of the heart in a manner still familiar in our modem colloquial language. In fact, many of our idioms related to the heart have their roots in the Bible. According to

Heart-Aches

Biblical tradition, the heart is clearly the center of the human being, around which everything else revolves. In a certain way, the Bible introduces its own language of the heart, which we will consider later. In any case, the Christian Holy Scriptures agree with the holy books of other religions in that they all state that love, hate, desire, passion, and sorrow all dwell in the heart. The Christian tradition has resolutely continued the emphasis on the heart as the center of man and his redemption, even developing some special aspects of this focus. The heart of Jesus became the central symbol of redemption, which is most often seen in the sacred art of the Mediterranean.

The movement of the *Sacred Heart of Jesus* has developed from the world of western monasteries, while the Heart Prayer has acquired an outstanding role in the Eastern Orthodox Church. The Catholics preserve the hearts of saints and worship them as relics. For example, Saint Teresa of Avila's heart has a special story connected with it. Saint Teresa reported in her writings that she had a powerful vision in which an angel pierced her heart with a glowing golden arrow. For some time after this vision, she was so ill that she could not leave her bed for months. Her heart has been preserved as a relic since 1582 and modern cardiologists found an infarct scar on it that could provide medical explanation of that visionary occurrence in the sixteenth century.

The movement of the *Sacred Heart of Jesus* reached its apex in the seventeenth century, with offshoots extending to our age today. An impressive body of documentation regarding the movement can be found in such places as the Sacre-Coeur (Sacred Heart) cathedral in Paris. Even as late as 1928, Pope Pius XI introduced the Festival of the Holy Heart. In addition, hundreds of prayers keep this form of heart symbolism in common usage today.

Throughout the ages, in religious writings as well as in folklore, the heart has remained the home of the emotions and the seat of the soul while its place in cultural history has experienced some fluctuations. Just as a pulse wave has its peaks and valleys, the pulse of the times also creates highs and lows in the appreciation of the heart and its role. At the beginning of our era, the young Christian movement, as the religion of love, was very close to the heart. However when the age of power politics began, this perspective did not last long. The recently persecuted Christians became the persecutors and naturally seemed more concerned with political power structures than listening to the voice of the heart. Because of this heartless attitude, the still young, but no longer innocent, Christian church smashed the movement of the Gnostics with cold-blooded harshness.

One thousand years later, the religion of the heart incarnated in the pure piety of the Cathari and Albigenses, who gained considerable influence. The epoch of the minnesingers had begun and with it came the poetry of courtly love—aimed at a purely spiritual-emotional form of love—and so once again the heart enjoyed a place of honor. King Solomon's *Song of Songs,* which seems to be a peculiar exception in the Bible, probably enjoyed better understanding then that at any other time. When even the Knights Templar began to place the feminine principle (in the form of Mary) in a central position, the established powers of state and church united their might to smash and denounce this movement of heartfelt love.

A similar situation occurred in more modern times when the Age of Enlightenment put an end to the Middle Ages by its emphasis upon reason, thereby suppressing everything emotional, including the role of the heart. At the turn of the nineteenth century, Romanticism once again celebrated a victory of the heart over reason. However, by the middle of the century, the time of the heart had passed once again. The scientific age had dawned and with it came a technological perspective, one which assigned a place to everything—particularly all matters of the heart. The basic attitude of science (strictly reason oriented) stimulated the brain tremendously, but it rapidly developed a heartless aspect as well. This has then naturally evolved into the compulsive structures by which we make our hearts and our lives callous and difficult today.

In comparison, the medical history of the heart is more modest—if we exclude the old, more esoteric medicine of antiquity and the shamanistic medicine of our ancestors. The history of cardiology, the medical science of the heart and its problems, first began with William Harvey (1578-1657) and his trailblazing discovery of blood circulation. However, the process used to make this discovery (and therefore the beginning of the scientific cardiovascular system) has a blemish that some people prefer to ignore. Harvey achieved his goal not through scientific hypotheses and corresponding experiments but through analogous deduction (the thinking method of esoteric tradition and religion, which is highly suspect to science). He called the heart "the original source of life and the sun of a small world," just as the sun deserves the name Heart of the World. This way of thinking is completely aligned with that of Paracelsus and is far removed from any form of scientific analysis in the modern sense. It was probably because of this perspective that the medical world was unable to accept Harvey's discovery for over two centuries. Even as recently as 1841, the famous Munich doctor Ringeis ridiculed Harvey's research, claiming that this theory had led the therapy of heart disease down the wrong track.

Only at the end of the nineteenth century did the rigid perspective of the medical profession find enlightenment. The Russian physician Korotkow (1874-1920) achieved a major step forward when he measured the pressure in the long-denied circulatory system with the help of the pneumatic cuff developed by the Italian Riva-Rocci[1] (1863-1937). Since then, the measurement of blood pressure has developed rapidly—perhaps the most rapid and impressive series of developments in the entire history of medicine. No other medical parameters are as frequently measured and as well established in the public consciousness as body temperature and blood pressure. Nearly every individual knows his or her blood pressure today. Even patients who cannot state their weight sometimes know these magical numbers. Today, many pharmacies have devices that automatically measure it and even several department stores feature such services. Medical doctors throughout the world make an unintended apology to Harvey every day by monitoring the circulatory system through blood pressure. This happens about one billion times a year in the United States alone.

We also monitor the heartbeat with great interest and increasingly sophisticated technology. We listen to it with stethoscopes and we examine the response of the needles on our echocardiographs and electrocardiogram machines. However, do we really understand the language of the heart better than we did before all of this technology? With all of this sophisticated equipment and apparent omnipotence, have we not forgotten the most simple and natural things? We can break open the calcareous constrictions of the coronary vessels with balloon catheters and control spasmodic constriction with nitroglycerin. A bypass can circumvent some narrow places, now that brilliant surgeons have learned how to move a piece of saphenous vein from the leg to the heart. We have become experts at exchanging a rundown heart for a fresh one and we have even developed machines that can temporarily take over the entire action of the heart.

If all else fails, a baboon must suffer as its heart is skillfully removed—or should we say *torn out*? Does *cut out* sound better? No, we prefer to say *operate!* We are truly brilliant at surgery on many levels. We have time, money, and the inclination for all of this. However, if a person wants to relieve his heavy heart, he can no longer find a doctor who will listen to him. A lack of time or money becomes an issue and, in the worst case, even a doctor has no interest in listening to him. We might as well admit it—the medical profession unerringly follows the way of progress and such progress is certainly not a path to the heart.

We can listen to the heart better than ever, but we no longer listen to what it has to say, we no longer understand its language. Patients probably still come to us with their heavy hearts, but we do not permit them—or they no longer desire—to pour them out to us. We should *want* to listen and to repair their hearts with them since even they themselves listen less and less to the heart, let alone obey it.

In order to obey one's own heart one must first learn to listen to it again. In addition to having the willingness to do so, one must also relearn the language of the heart if one is to understand its message. Medical technology can merely help one become more familiar with the technical aspects of the heart, serving in a reasonable, cold-blooded, and even heartless way. In order to learn how to understand the true language of the heart, there is nothing one needs more that is more important than one's own heart—vast and open.

A school of psychosomatic medicine was already in existence during the first half of the twentieth century, inspired by a form of psychoanalysis which accepted the language of the organs and the heart. Georg Groddeck made a particularly significant contribution as a "shaman in doctor's clothes." However, this approach broke down when innovative medications promised to treat all afflictions in a much simpler and seemingly more direct manner. Our basic attitude—enslaved as it is by science—tends naturally to prefer a shallow approach, whereby we rely on symptomatic remedies and so avoid the center (or heart) of the real problems.

Today, there is evidence of a new movement to change our ways and so openness to the heart and its concerns will once again be possible. We can learn from the past and hopefully we won't repeat our extreme behavior, forsaking one path wholesale for another. Perhaps we can retain our reasoned and scientific results when we venture forward into the depths of a holistic point of view. However, at least in certain phases, cool reason will have to be silenced in order to make room for the personal logic of myth, folk wisdom, and the pictorial language of the Bible. This should be somewhat easier after our excursion into the history of the heart. As we have seen, science has only shown interest in the heart for a short period of time while, on the other hand, mythology, poetry, folk medicine, and the esoteric disciplines can look back on millennia of tradition. Why should they not be in a position to offer something deeper and more essential but definitely of at least equal value?

I wish for both the reader and for myself, the open-mindedness and sense of adventure required when it comes to attentively listening to the language of the heart. Before we find our way into the inner world and the world of the heart, here are a few considerations to help pave the way.

4.

Symptoms as an Expression of Inner Reality

4.1 Evaluation of Symptoms

We intend to give credit to the heart in a far more extensive manner than orthodox medicine permits but without ignoring its research results. Therefore, we must view these results openly and without reservation. Then, if we wish to use such thoroughly researched symptomatic descriptions for our purposes, our first important step is to detach ourselves from science's usual approach of evaluation or devaluation. According to accepted practice, a symptom represents a bad, unpleasant defect of one's organism, having struck the body because of some unfortunate mistake within ourselves or within our environment, and so we should eliminate this defect as quickly as possible.

However, rather than simply wishing to eliminate this fault, we want to work with it. We even want it to teach us what we are *missing*. Removed from its negative connotation, the symptom can become a guide on our path, helping us in our development. Just as we normally team up with the doctor against the symptom, we can also put ourselves on the side of the symptom.

From such a perspective, we can investigate what our problem is or what it is that we are missing. This is why when a doctor poses the question, "What is the problem?" patients always answer with a description of their symptoms (since these can best reveal the missing principle).

Furthermore, we can exonerate the term *symptom* by noting that each human being—without exception—has symptoms. Therefore, it is not a question of whether or not symptoms are present but it is merely an issue of their severity. With this perspective, it is then just a small step to the insight that every person is sick—a fact that all religions proclaim.[2]—In order to improve one's personal situation, the human being urgently needs the Redeemer since she is unredeemed or not whole. This idea hides behind the teachings of original sin. The phrase "to commit a sin" might be the key since sin originally derives from the Greek word that means "to separate" and "to miss the point." The philosophy behind this word implies that our birth into this world of opposites leads us to feel isolated from the Unity—or, expressed in different terms, we have "missed the point." Almost all cultures consider "the point" to be the symbol of unity. This becomes particularly clear with respect to the central point of a mandala. Even in mathematics, the point is a non-dimensional symbol.

With this understanding, the idea of sin could lose something of its moralizing assessment. As denizens of this polarized world that splits into opposites, we have all separated from the Unity— the original state of Paradise—and therefore we are all isolated or sinful. This is neither unjust nor terrible but is, on the contrary, necessary for our development. This polarity in the world of opposites is the counter-part to unity and our only chance for true self-realization. Yet, understanding is required conscious to find the way back to unity. Our polarized consciousness cannot comprehend the Unity and depends constantly on contrasts. We would not know what high is without low. Poor would be meaningless without rich. Each of our ideas only has meaning through its counterpart. Such opposites are as dependent on one another as the two sides of a coin. Knowledge of the whole in such a polarized[3] world requires familiarity with both poles. Otherwise, knowledge is not possible. In Paradise, Eve's nibbling at the fruit of the Tree of Knowledge (of Good and Evil) was therefore not a terrible mistake but the beginning of the evolutionary path. It was an error perhaps, but a necessary one since it helped gain what was missing—knowledge. This error led to a world of opposites—into isolation from the unity of Paradise.

We are sinners, we are isolated from unity—we all have symptoms—and within a polarity there is no other way.

4.2 Symptoms as Companions on the Path

In practical terms, we must admit to ourselves that symptoms have always been—at the very least—companions to us. We carry them with us through life, whether we value them or not. Many people suffer their company for decades without questioning their actual purpose. Experience on the part of psychotherapy proves that such a dismissive attitude does not simplify life but actually makes it more difficult. On our journey through life we collect many things and take them with us. We want to possess as much as possible, the ideal being to possess everything, and we believe that this will make us happy. The lives of world leaders and the immensely rich prove that this idea is an illusion. Despite this fact, many people strive for wholeness and completion by making as much of the world as possible their own physical possessions. If they had to give up some of these possessions without some form of compensation, they would feel that they missed them. The situation regarding symptoms that we have collected on our journey through life is quite similar. We would also miss them as part of our wholeness if we had to give them up without an acceptable replacement, which is why most people cling to their symptoms as they would to a valued possession. Our striving for wholeness or perfection has set its roots too deep for us simply to release it.

Just as our desire to buy a house often indicates that we are missing a home of our own, the acquisition of a symptom indicates that we have missed this (principle). Until now, it may not have been the right time for this particular theme in our life, but when the time is ripe, we buy the house or come down with the symptom. Both of these cases are a blessing, albeit the latter is more difficult to understand. On the basis of daily life experience we know that the ownership of a house can become a burden, while a symptom can become a blessing if it opens the patient's eyes to something of significance, or if it radically changes the course of a life at a decisive moment. Every doctor knows at least some patients who are grateful for their heart attack because of what they were able to learn as a result of it. Once again, it is merely a question of value. Unfortunately, our society projects a very one-sided response against heart attack. However, this common view of such symptoms is not the only way to see them. Many native peoples who live in close harmony with nature are familiar with diseases of initiation, for which they often practically yearn. A person can only become a shaman, for example, when a corresponding course of disease initiates him. Until recently, even in our culture people recognized the great importance of certain puerile diseases for childhood development.

Whatever our attitude is towards symptoms, they are comrades on our path and are much more difficult to get rid of than all of our material possessions. Yes, they are about as difficult to get rid of as a shadow on a sunny day—and this fact has its deeper reason. Through simple tricks, one can shake off the shadow by running out of the sunshine. However, as soon as one returns to the light, one meets the shadow again. The situation is very similar with symptoms. Suppressive medications can help to push them aside for a while—this is just as popular as it is profitable. The symptom shifts from organ to organ and the patient goes from specialist to specialist. Yet, if one views this in the light of a corresponding far-reaching therapy, the symptom may perhaps change its outer form, but its message has not changed. This is true because the symptom is the expression of our inner shadow.

4.3 "Causes" of Symptoms

Consideration of the topic of the shadow leads to a critical perspective for both psychological and medical questions. One can only overlook this decision point if it is limited to a very superficial phenomenological level, which frequently occurs in orthodox medicine and psychology. There, one assumes that certain symptoms strike us by simple coincidence, with pathogens perhaps hiding behind them, but that they bear no deeper meaning. Because of one's own self-imposed limits, one does not ask the deeper questions and so the true meaning remains hidden and treatment does not go past the superficial description of the symptoms and their therapy. If one has an interest in the meaning of the symptoms and their language, one is sure to discover something of interest, although orthodox science has branded such a process as unscientific.

However, measured by the standards of knowledge for modern physics, the accusation of being unscientific applies most severely to orthodox medicine itself. The science of physics has evolved in such a way that the principle of causality—the basis of natural sciences—has been reduced to an absurd extreme, to the point where it has deprived the common understanding of natural science of its very basis. Today, physicists can prove that causality does not exist and that an inexplicable synchronicity rules us instead. The result is that because they have always and exclusively looked for causes in the past, orthodox medicine and psychology are missing a base.

For better or for worse, we will have to continue to deal with causality in our models of the world—just as we assume that there is such a thing as absolute time, despite Einstein having established its relative nature. However, since physics thinks of causality in relative terms, there is no longer a reason to place the old school's understanding of causality above everything else, which was never the case in everyday life anyway. We say, for example, "I am arriving now because I left home one hour ago." This reasoning (causality) is correct in terms of common science because the cause (leaving home) lies in the past. However, we also say in the same way, "I have to go now because in two hours I have to be in San Francisco." Here, the cause (to have to be in San Francisco) lies in the future, and this would be a forbidden causality in terms of common science. A simple example can clarify the limitations of this approach, which many universities vehemently preach, even today, in the age of modern physics.

Let us consider any type of moving process, such as a well-known game—soccer for example—in a scientific manner. The first difficulty in its examination results from the complexity of the game. Because living processes are so complex, they easily overtax science, which must cut small sections out of a whole situation in order to analyze it in detail. The human being as a whole is too extensive to be viewed in detail in a single glance and so the preferred approach is to look at each human being piece by piece. This technique of 'divide and conquer' endangers science's ability to see life for what it is.

While analyzing the soccer game, we also must proceed in a similar manner and single out a short maneuver—for example, a penalty kick situation. The ball lies on the penalty spot as a forward runs up and kicks the ball. We select this moment and ask the standard scientific question. "Why—why does the forward kick the ball?" Next we must investigate many penalty situations in order to discover the reason. This is not easy since nothing remains constant—a different player always runs up and always kicks a different ball. The referees change as often as the field, the spectators, and the stadium. A foul (but never the same one) often precedes the situation while sometimes only a handled ball caused the penalty. Ultimately, after much research, one discovers the single consistent and reproducible cause for the penalty kick—the referee's whistle. Only the whistle is common to all penalty kicks and nothing happens without it.

A feeling of unease may creep up behind us when we consider this analysis, as it does for an increasing number of people when they consider scientific medicine. Somehow, the essential nature of soccer has eluded us in this analysis. There are other, if less scientific, reasons for the penalty kick. For example, one could name the desire to score a goal. However, this cause lies in the future. One could possibly find another reason in the rules of the game—the pattern of it, meaning that many games have been played before and many penalty kicks have occurred. Therefore, the player surely moves within a prescribed pattern. A rather banal yet important reason also lies in the material manifestations of the ball, the field, and the other essential physical elements of the game. Three further reasons have now joined the analytic one. In Greek antiquity, people already worked quite successfully with these four causes. For them—and for many cultures before them—every occurrence, and therefore every symptom of illness as well, had a purpose that pointed to the future and to a pattern that made it understandable.

Measured in terms of reality—as revealed by modem physics today and known by esoteric tradition since time immemorial—it is Just as valid to seek a meaning that lies in the future as it is to ask for a cause (such as a pathogen) that has its origin in the past. Both are equally helpful intellectual constructions, although neither one corresponds to the complete reality, they both find justification because each one helps us to better understand the overall picture of a symptom.

4.4 Medical Principle of the Conservation of Energy and Its Shadow

If we consider symptoms as pictures or patterns, and if we search for their significance, we will always find a correlation in meaning within the life of the patient. The symptom depicts an element that the patient does not consciously want to perceive in his life, which is why one reacts so strongly against otherwise medically harmless symptoms like warts and pimples. This is not surprising. The suppressed parts of consciousness spread throughout the body and become visible to everyone. At the same time, they use the body as a stage for a play that one did not want to see, or hear, or even admit to oneself However, now one is forced to feel it.

From physics we know that nothing can simply disappear. The only possibility is to transmute one form into another—such as ice into water or steam. In this example, the condition of the ice (which is water's most material condition) embodies the least energy. Energy—thermal energy—must enter the situation in order to achieve a liquid state and more energy (for example, during cooking) is necessary to reach the even more energetic gaseous state. Physicists would say that the vibration of the molecules becomes increasingly active from ice through to steam, which means that the molecules vibrate with increasing frequency. In the opposite direction, from steam, to water, to ice, the molecular vibrations decrease their kinetic rate and energy escapes from the water.

All things considered, in these transformation processes energy can neither be greater nor disappear. It remains constant. Physics knows this as the principle of conservation of energy. Interestingly enough. Depth Psychology is also familiar with these so- called aggregate states. The solid state (ice) symbolizes matter. The earthly component, and consequently the body. The liquid state (water) represents the emotional element, while the gaseous state (steam) can be taken as a metaphor for spiritual energy. Esoteric psychology follows physics even further in that it also acknowledges the different vibratory levels from matter, to soul, to spirit. The result of these concepts—and most importantly the experience of many psychotherapists—is that nothing disappears in the realm of the living. Again, transformation is the only possibility. One can also assume that the law of conservation of energy exists in the realm of the living as well. Therefore, emotional energy can very well be transmuted into physical form and vice versa, but it will never disappear.

Each of us is familiar with the connection between these various levels from our day-to-day experiences. When a suggestive Joke evokes an emotion that develops against one's conscious will, the facial skin blushes. The heart may pound in joy or expectation and we can develop cold feet due to fear. A swallowed rage can also turn into gastritis. The inflamed mucous coat of the stomach (the symptom) leads to an obvious conclusion about the unexpressed emotion resulting from the suppression (swallowing) of rage.

Therefore, a theme can materialize from the body to consciousness and thereby shift to the spiritual level—if the necessary energy is provided. In this way the problem is liberated from its physical existence, which corresponds to an aspect of the shadow because the consciousness for the theme behind it is lacking. For example, energy in the form of psychotherapy or meditation, when applied to a symptom, establishes the relationship to the emotional level and almost instantly the body seems relieved. However, now the soul is suffering.

In a further step, one could raise the theme to the spiritual level (again with considerable effort) so that the pattern behind it becomes recognizable and—above all—accepted in all its depth. In this case, the theme is on the highest level of energy, relieving body and soul. However, the consciousness must now become involved directly with the theme.

This can be—and usually is—quite unpleasant. If this were not so, the patient would not have suppressed it in the first place. If one works through this theme and finally resolves it, the energy still does not vanish. In an ideal situation, one consciously sends it to where it originally belonged.

In short, one could view the example of a gastric ulcer in the following way. The first step is to re-experience all of the swallowed emotions—this replaces physical pain with emotional pain. The next step is to realize that these emotions are quite justified and correct, but that they were merely located in an unsuitable place. It then becomes possible to direct them at their real target, such as the boss, the partner, or some other responsible antagonist. (Later in this book, angina pectoris is used as an example to show how a concrete transformation, from the level of the body to consciousness, and the corresponding principles have solidified into the material state of the body.)

Therefore, everything is perpetually preserved, while only its appearance changes. One can see this in the example of water appearing in its liquid state, its solid ice aspect, and its gaseous form as steam. The essential nature always remains in these transformations—even if one may not discover the connection between the water on earth and the clouds in the sky at first glance. Only a child, who is not yet familiar with the physical correlations, could claim that evaporated water has vanished into nothingness, without substitution.

Decades have passed since C. G. Jung introduced the concept of the shadow to the field of psychology, a theory which occurred to him after he perceived that nothing disappears within human life. Rather, it usually turns to the shadow side and so can become suppressed in the unconscious mind. Consequently, the unconscious belongs to us in a similar way that steam belongs to water. In the same manner that steam forms clouds and returns to earth as rain, the displaced elements also return from the human unconscious when a suitable opportunity arises. Dreams are one such opportunity; the symptoms of the body are another.

These reflect a part of the shadow that is ripe for the conscious mind. They emerge from the unconscious underworld's darkness onto the stage of the body, manifesting the simple evidence which a syndrome needs to become public—it needs attention. The symptoms send their message in a symbolic script that first needs deciphering—somewhat similar to dreams which illustrate the unconscious in symbolic, often mysterious and even paradoxical forms. At first glance, this might resemble some kind of indecipherable code. However, it is never wise to ignore it—no one can crack any code in the world by ignoring and suppressing it.

In order to learn to understand the language of symptoms, it is necessary to have a conscious, intuitive understanding of their symbolic world—full of apparent contradictions and logical inconsistencies. Contrasts in this world are often unusually close to one another—sometimes they even touch. Once a person is open to this perspective, things that seemed irreconcilable move closer together. Once one recognizes patterns rather than rationally analyzing connections on a shallow level, many things become clear. This applies not only to the realm of dreams and the world of symptoms but it also encompasses the rest of life. A person who thinks in purely rational terms will only feel astonished when, out of the blue, a peaceful demonstration deteriorates into a violent brawl. Only then might one realize the common theme that both sides are expressing in their violence. War and peace are two sides of the same coin. We suddenly stop wondering why some extremely committed environmentalists create very unpleasant fumes from their hand rolled cigarettes. The moral apostle and the porno fan, the criminologist and the criminal, the missionary and the aggressive atheist, the teetotaler and the alcoholic all share a common theme and are, therefore, much closer to one another than they, and a rational observer, might otherwise assume.

Symptoms are always reliable. They show with inexorable honesty the theme at hand. They are signals, signposts of the shadow, and everything that reaches a position of excessive importance in life can become a symptom. A person may denounce pornography at every opportunity or he may have an addictive desire for it. Both of these conditions demonstrate that a person is stuck. The difference is merely that the porno fan confronts his problem directly, while the moral apostle fights it via his projection onto others. From this perspective, the former could even be viewed as the more honest of the two.

4.5 Form and Meaning

Understanding the connection between form and meaning is another important step on the path towards uncovering the meaning of symptoms. In our modem times we have become accustomed to neglecting meaning for the sake of form. Our age has permitted many venerable, living rituals to stiffen into habits, leaving them to lead a shadowy existence as dead hulks, devoid of meaning. The lives of the ancients were full of ritual and purpose, while our lives seem to be full of habits and material possessions. However, now everything has lost its meaning. A striking example is orthodox medicine, which has achieved indisputable success in research concerning form but which has, however, become quite blind to its purpose in the process.

In light of our metaphor of the body as a stage on which the explosive theme of symptom plays in the manner of a drama, let us take a scientific look at such a play. Such an analysis would result in a precise listing of all of the materials used to create the scenery and props. We would record the number, sex, body weight, size, and skin color of the actors as well as the fabric and color of their costumes. We would note the length of their lines—the count of their words even to the very letter. We would measure the volume of the acoustics and we might set the intensity of the lighting in the individual scenes precisely and to every increment. As long as we continued to analyze in this manner, we would certainly not come any closer to the meaning of the play—to its essential nature.

In many places today, we overestimate the value of form while neglecting meaning. However, one must also be careful not to devalue form entirely. On the contrary, form represents the best way to come into contact with meaning. However, form by itself becomes meaningless or, expressed in other terms, anything not assigned a meaning remains meaningless. Orthodox medicine has collected valuable information about form and we must make grateful use of this information for our purposes, in order to draw conclusions about the meaning from this form.

If we consider the symptoms in their physical form, the props and costumes that they have borrowed from the body, we will find indications of the emotional meaning expressed within them. The stage (the body) is very important in this respect—just as the theater and its stage is the medium needed to express the meaning of a play to its audience, the body is our contact point with the meaning of the symptom.

4.6 The Daily Pact with the Devil

Symptoms are something deeply human and are grounded in a basic human attitude—avoiding pain while searching for pleasure. In earlier times, when someone focused her consciousness with much more intense energy on the *Other World,* the consciousness was also correspondingly more open to the unavoidable suffering and difficult lessons of our world. The life and suffering of Christ played an exemplary role in this regard while the teachings of Buddha still play such a role for other cultural groups. One of the principles of Buddha's teachings is that everything that has come into existence is suffering.

As the orientation towards this world increased in the West, the tendency to avoid any type of discomfort accompanied it, and became even more prominent with the tendency to reject themes related to suffering and exertion. This process overlooks the fact that one cannot keep the inevitable at bay forever and that it will certainly never go away entirely. The only way of eliminating a problem is to solve it. Even when a problem has been tackled, it has not really disappeared forever. Instead, it has moved on to another, perhaps less trying level. Each of us has many such steps of liberation behind us. For example, we all learned how to solve the problem of learning to read back in elementary school. However, this did not mean that the task of reading no longer existed for us, but it had stopped being a problem. Had we not learned how to read back then, reading would still be a very urgent issue for us today, as our daily activities would revolve around our illiteracy and strategies to compensate for it.

Today we entertain the notion that something removed is really gone—vanished—dissolved into nothingness. However, it has only been displaced, as the word *re-moved* clearly shows US, and therefore continues to exist. As we have already noted, the principle of energy conservation also applies between the emotional and the physical levels. Because of a lack of appreciation for this law, a typical human situation results, as illustrated in Goethe's legend of Doctor Faust, a story which has been repeated millions of times since its first telling. Faust wanted to achieve the Ultimate Knowledge at any price and, in vain, he had hoped to receive such knowledge from science. For this reason, he turned to the Lord of this World—Mephistopheles.[4] As a pledge, Faust offered Mephistopheles his soul, which apparently meant less to him at that moment than this final knowledge, and so he enjoyed his power over Mephistopheles' world of opposites. However, when it finally came time to pay, he turned a deaf ear and, as his creditor, Mephistopheles was forced to threaten compulsory measures. The path of Faust's development—now essentially at its beginning—consisted of liberation or redemption from his debt in this pact. To keep his soul, he could no longer afford any form of stagnation as he had to consciously continue his development step by step and so bring light into the dark realms of his being.

In the same manner as Faust, we barter for our symptoms. We want to achieve our desires "at any price" and then avoid dealing with our pain, also "at any price." Let us examine a common example. We want to achieve power, become the boss, and thereby avoid being helpless and at someone else's mercy. Without admitting to ourselves what kind of pact we have made, we begin to slave and toil. We will pay "any price" to suppress this choice from our consciousness and then, when it is time to pay and the price presents itself (manifesting, for example, as prematurely ruined physical and emotional health), we turn a deaf ear and do not want to pay the piper. We inevitably have the same choice as Faust. We may try to refuse, but if we do we will pay for this game of blind man's bluff with a loss of awareness in the corresponding regions of the soul, and so suffer under the accompanying symptoms on the level of the body. On the other hand, we can choose Faust as our example and set out on an arduous path of development, one that means consciously recognizing the pact, accepting it, and learning from it, or from its implications.

4.7 Symptoms—A Summary

1. This work is not concerned with any particular system of values, but rather with an interpretation—even if the language used is often and necessarily judgmental.
2. Everyone has symptoms since everyone is unhealthy. We are all sick (sinful) as we live isolated from the Unity in a world of opposites—in a state of polarity.
3. This state of opposites is necessary for our knowledge and for our path to becoming conscious human beings.
4. Every symptom is a 'mistake' in the sense that it shows us that something is missing. The value system behind this symptom (or error) is relative and its condition depends on a particular time and culture.
5. Nothing in the spiritual-emotional sphere can utterly disappear, in the same way that nothing can disappear in the material-physical realm either. The very farthest it can go is to sink into the unconscious mind (the shadow) for a while.
6. Form and meaning belong together. The form is the necessary point of contact to the meaning.

7. A symptom results from the compulsory execution of a pact that one has voluntarily entered into and, in this respect, it is both consistent and honest. It is the conscious redemption of this debt or sin that makes a person whole.

By keeping these seven steps in mind, we will succeed in releasing symptoms from their "demonic" interpretation and so prevent ourselves from sulking at our lot in life. Instead of denigrating our symptoms as one of the unfortunate cruelties of life, we can return to the wise approach of letting them be our guides.

5.

The Language of the Heart in the Bible

There is probably no better source for becoming familiar with language related to the heart than the Bible. One may even consider it a dictionary in this respect. It refers to the heart as the center, the pivotal point, and the most important concern. Frequently, the heart is even used to represent the entire human being. Expressions such as "until his heart trusts," "with hope in the heart," "when sorrow touches the heart," or "giving the heart confidence," refers to the human being as a whole. When God admonishes humans to "guard their hearts," He means that they should be cautious.

There are many places in the Bible where the heart clearly represents the entire person. It often emphasizes the heart as the decisive place in the human being—the cardinal point around which everything else revolves. It is the place that represents the Unity and the divinity within each of us. This is why God demands that we turn to Him with heart and soul—not half-heartedly. When we make sacrifices to Him, we should do so without duplicity (undivided hearts). He wants us to seek Him with simplicity in the heart and He does not want us to pray to Him with a conflicted heart. The heart as the place of unity does not tolerate any dualism in the figurative sense. When we speak to Him, God expects that we will carry our hearts on our sleeves and He does not expect us to speak with forked tongues in the manner of the snake in the Garden of Eden. With this honesty, which comes from the center (more precisely, from the heart), we should consecrate our hearts to Him.

The Bible leaves no doubt that God's kingdom of heaven—which Christ describes as being within us—opens up within the heart. "My heart is joyful in the Lord." It is the center of our existence. Desiring God from the heart means that we love Him from our depths. This leads to the heart as the symbolic starting point for love. Biblical examples of this are numerous and they illustrate clearly the differences between the love of the human ego and the love of the higher self—so-called divine love. The Bible therefore warns about the desires of the heart, in the sense that the heart can let itself be deluded by objects of desire. In the eyes of God, the deluded heart apparently lets one appear foolish "in whose heart dwells nothing but foolishness." The Bible suggests that one "turns one's heart to God " "turns it towards Him," "inclines it towards Him," and as a response one should "let one's heart be touched by Him." One should "prepare one's heart for Him," "take Him into the heart," and "not be unfaithful" to one's heart, nor should one "let it be stolen." One also addresses God accordingly; "Lord, my heart is wax in your hands." "Help me so that my heart does not stray from you." The Bible also states the following sentiment very well: "where your treasure is, your heart will also be" and so it recommends not to "hang one's heart on Just anything," but rather to open it to God—to make Him one's treasure. Obeying Him from one's whole heart means to listen to Him from within the heart and to allow His words to be the nourishment of the heart. The Bible lays the corner stone for the goal of this development as it is divine love from a pure heart. "Blessed are those who are pure of heart."

God will measure us by this goal: "However, the Lord looks into the heart." He knows that He has planted eternity into the heart. At the proper time He will see what a person has made

Heart-Aches

of it—whether or not one has become receptive to what He has set in the heart. Then He will come to search the person's heart and examine their heart and soul.[5]

As the center represents the entire person and the core of love, the heart is also the highest sensory organ and the place of deepest feeling, with its ability extending far beyond the five physical senses. We often describe the heart as deeply moved, happy, fearful, or sad. It can feel comforted, refreshed, full of worry, frightened, ill-tempered, and blinded.

When the heart can no longer understand what it must perceive or bear, what it must see, it begins to lament figuratively—even worse, to bleed on an emotional level. If it has turned away from the divine principle and from love, it will gradually close up (constrict) and become increasingly numb. Defiant, unruly, haughty, and false—it may utterly dry up or wither. Such an obstinate heart is then naturally cold, rigid, and utterly and completely sealed. The end has also come for the heart as a sensory organ—it becomes insensitive and hard as a stone, as the patient becomes someone resembling a heartless person.

Finally, the Bible also purports the heart to be an important organ of expression. God can perceive and evaluate a person through the heart's various manifestations. The Bible speaks of "all of the heart's thoughts and efforts." Here the heart is joyful and exultant and in good spirits. The heart runs over, wells up, sweeps a person away, becomes disloyal, and begins to hate. The Bible mentions "the senses of the heart" and "losing heart." One heart feels contempt, another even hates. Some hearts bend under the troubles of life while others bow down in humility. Hearts become agitated, seek violence and revenge, or allow themselves to be tempted to go astray by money. There are cunning and treacherous hearts and there are hearts whose owners make them into "a den of thieves." The biblical tradition also views the heart as the cosmic clock when it states, "The heart proclaims the hour to the people."

The heart, as our center, is also the arena of the steps of main conflict and development. Just as one can love God in one's heart, according to the Bible one can also commit adultery there. Any type of distress eats away at the heart, and fear and sorrow touch the heart. According to the Bible, the most noble sentiments have their starting point here, and this is also where malicious glee erupts in its various forms. Here is where one believes, doubts, and contemplates one's most secret intentions, where one lets the Christ come in, and where one cherishes people and objects that are truly close to one's heart. "It breaks my heart" signifies genuine emotion and expression. When one "washes the heart pure" one can expect to be truly clean thereafter. Such action makes room in the heart for those that are very special to us. When one "opens the heart," one is completely open, just as any action that one makes "from the heart" is carried through to completion. If one "keeps God in the heart," then God fills a person absolutely. "The Lord keep holy in your hearts," "until the morning star rises in your hearts."

6.

The Heart in Timeless Words

If one considers expressions of colloquial language—proverbs and familiar quotations concerned with the heart—it is immediately obvious that the heart appears in a manner analogous to that of the Bible. One is dealing with an archetypal understanding of the heart and, although it has little in common with the medical perspective, it is quite consistent with it on many other levels. Language becomes an important aid. The philosopher Heidegger very aptly said, "Language conceals the treasure of all that is essential within itself." It expresses the central principle of the heart from time immemorial when it speaks of "the light of life that lives in the heart" or even of the "light of the heart that is the center of a human being." One should also mention the venerable idea of the "sphere of light that sinks into the heart," as well as the "spark of the soul" that the mystics claim dwells within the heart. "Whatever you set your heart on, your God is also there," said Martin Luther; he was somewhat more oriented towards the outer world.

Folk wisdom very clearly addresses the issue of the hierarchy of the heart and the brain, in contrast with the approach of orthodox medicine. In order to evaluate a person, you must look into his heart and not into his mind. The Chinese culture says that if you want to test a person, the most important thing to verify is whether he has a heart (Li Yii). In *The Death of Wallenstein*, Schiller writes, "the heart and not his opinion honors the man." Blaise Pascal says, "It is the heart that experiences God and not the mind." Goethe called the heart the "youngest, most diverse, most flexible, most changeable, and most easily shaken part of Creation." A common German saying reports, "If one steals someone's heart, the mind offers no defense." It is understandable that the question of whether someone "has their heart in the right place" is quite important. Its location in the center of the body is obvious and so it should also be the core of life. In this context comes a further quote from Pascal, "The heart has its reason that the mind does not know."

Another bit of German folk wisdom expresses the dangers that threaten when the emphasis has shifted to the mind, "The heart dries up when the mind rules by itself." The following sentences come from Saint Hildegard of Bingen, who saw the heart as the *domus animae* (the house of the soul). These words teach us the proper relationship between the two centers:

> The soul is like a fire at the center of the dwelling. The thoughts come from there and spread up into the mind, where they are reshaped. Only together with the coldness of the brain does the fire of the heart result in the harmony of thoughts.

Theodor Fontane had a similar perspective, "Oh learn to think with the heart and learn to feel with the mind." Consequently, we have adages that convey the idea of teaching the heart, a topic we too frequently cast aside in the curriculum of our modem schools and universities. No wonder the heart cries for attention and care. It is also no wonder that we hardly ever "speak from the heart" or even from "heart to heart" anymore. Our education concentrates in the brain or in our ability to use our hands. We speak with a "sharp tongue" and a "brilliant mind" and, if necessary, also with our "hands and feet."

Heart-Aches

Yet, the heart lies fallow and uneducated; it may even be *locked.* We seem to have lost the "key to the heart." Language also reveals how we can find it once again, "Through love, all things that the mind considered too difficult can become easier" (a Persian proverb). "The angels call it heavenly joy; the devils call it hellish suffering; the people call it love," (Heinrich Heine). According to folk wisdom, the proverbial "secret of the heart" lies in love. The yearning of the heart strives to *unite* with other hearts until we are "one heart and one soul." The "house of the heart" readily opens up to a chance for love and it lets in anything or anyone who is a stranger. The two *houses* become one, as the two souls become one: "Hearts find each other." There is no state on earth that more closely approaches the unity of Paradise and, therefore, it is the goal of human longing. When the heart opens up to another person, to everyone and to everything (and thereby to God), it achieves the goal—the "simplicity of the heart."

This is the state that mystics strive for. For example, Meister Eckehart described this goal in the following words, "The eye with which I look at God is the eye with which God looks at me." He is one with everything and everything is one with Him and within Him. The heart is *open,* and it is so *wide* that it includes the entirety of Creation. People in love can see the reflection of this encompassing love, as they feel an expansive desire to embrace the entire world. "Nothing is difficult for he who loves," said Cicero. "Love remains the golden ladder on which the heart climbs to heaven," is an old German proverb. The following idea from Dostoyevski is also pertinent: "To love a person means to see him as God meant him to be seen."

On the human level of our polarized world, the Unity is usually quite distant—or as Schopenhauer expressed it, "All of life is ambiguous." Without a doubt, opposites characterize life in our polarity, while it is precisely love that permits us a glance at the Unity time and again. Also, the heart is the place where a glance can penetrate the narrow borders of a world ruled by reason. Language then becomes the virtual symbol of love, ranging from the divine love of God, to the love joining two people, to the one that is effective in advertising (for instance, "I <3 New York"). One decorates one's vehicle with a heart sticker and lovers scratch their names, framed with a heart, into the trunk of a tree. The symbol of the heart always represents an individual person's longing to experience the Unity while still living in a duality.

The two upper curves of the symbolic heart merge into a point as our glance automatically gravitates to this point. A symbol of human love is often a valentine pierced by Cupid's arrow. As the son of Venus, the goddess of love, Cupid, the god of love blindly but unerringly shoots the hearts of human beings to set their hearts ablaze. Sometimes Cupid even sets a torch to the unsuspecting victim's hearts. The people struck by these arrows of love immediately feel as if they are on fire; when they feel inflamed with burning passion for one another, this is perfectly understandable. Hot love lets its flames blaze up and rage in these *burning* hearts. Some time ago, teenagers referred to their sweethearts as their "flame." However, all of this deals with a very human and therefore polarized form of love. After all, in order to realize the concerns of his mother—Venus, the goddess of love—Cupid uses the weapons of his father—Mars, the god of war. As a result, this type of fiery love is very polarized, as it has more to do with the diametrically opposed sexuality of two people ablaze for each other than it has to do with the heart's center. Cupid's Greek name, *Eros,* is more fitting since eroticism is the primary factor involved here.

Sayings such as my "Queen of Hearts," or its counterpart the "Jack of Hearts," reveal the central (heart) significance of the affected person. The people that one clasps to one's heart are those whom one really likes. As the next step in a committed relationship, one offers one's heart and therefore oneself. When one loses one's heart to someone, the victim of love is practically without his own center and, therefore, the smitten person is far removed from egocentrism and egoism. This type of feeling causes one to simply forget all rational arguments about a love that bridges deep chasms. A modern saying sums up the situation: "Love stimulates the heart while it numbs the mind." When someone with a crush obeys the heart and its language, the mind is outvoted; "Love is blind."

In the case when someone becomes attached to another, the object of love is "close to their heart." In a literal sense, these same words can describe the relationship between an unborn child and its mother. Although this image may not have much meaning anatomically, it is quite pertinent as a symbol for the relationship between mother and child. A relationship is usually very significant if it has evolved so that a friend becomes as close to a person's heart as one's own child. It is no coincidence that language has applied these expressions to the most important things in life.

In contrast, when something *touches* the heart, it moves the individual to his very depths. It is rare for something to weigh heavily on the heart (and therefore make the person "heavy-hearted"). Whatever pulls on the *heartstrings* reaches the heart—the center. Whatever one "takes to heart" is an experience that is likely to mark indelibly ones very depths. When a person wants to memorize something, he learns it "by heart."

If one *takes something to heart,* one finds it very important and the *heart's desire* is the deepest wish one can have, since it comes forth from the center. Similarly, the *joys of the heart* are also the deepest. "That warms the very cockles of my heart!" is a common English expression. If one wants another to speak truly from the core of his being—from his heart—one appeals to the other person's honor and honesty by asking him to place his *hand on his heart.* When connected to his center, a person can only speak the truth, *coming from a pure heart.*

In addition to its symbolism as the central point of the human being and the seat of love, the phrasing of language also reveals the heart as the most important sensory organ as well as the organ from which expression arises. This means that we *can feel, perceive, hear,* and *see* with the heart. Saint-Exupery's *The Little Prince* discloses, for example, that one can only see well with the heart, while the essential things remain invisible to the outer eyes. The heart is much more *sensitive* than all the other sensory organs and is, therefore, our most vulnerable organ. It is possible that not only bullets, knives, and spears can strike the heart, but words and barbed phrases also have the most effective power to wound the heart. Opponents will often fire entire (word) salvos directed at the heart. Also, because words can injure, such strikes can also cause damage in the long term. A heart that has suffered emotional hurt often enough will ultimately become physically sick as well.

However, before we discuss the signs of illness, we should take a close look at the language of everyday life as this will tell us how the heart deals with, and reacts to, various sensory stimuli. To express elation one says, "My heart is pounding with joy." It can *leap within* when excitement or joy is too great and the heart can even *burst* with pride or with happiness. This danger is particularly important when joy surprises and overwhelms one at the same time. The heart may then react with a shock and can even *stop* when the person is startled. An event that hits "like a bolt out of the blue" can be too strong for the heart and its rhythm, as it overwhelms the victim and her heart. In milder cases and, above all, in situations associated with excitement, one's heart can respond to such encounters with a galloping rhythm or even a sensation of fluttering. This could even signify heart fibrillation (once again, medical science makes a connection).

If a surprise is mixed with fear, the victim may feel the same way as expressed by the idiom: "My heart sank down into my boots." Such a fallen heart is naturally in a conceivably bad position for facing the cause of the fear with impunity. It would be much more appropriate to handle a fearful situation in the manner expressed in the following idioms: "I took up my heart in my two hands" or "1 took heart." These two phrases describe a person with a strong heart—with the courage to face up to a situation.

Courage also resides in the heart, as does its opposite—cowardice. A *brave heart* or a *heart like a lion* distinguishes a courageous person, hence the epithet of Richard the Lionheart. On the other hand, it is well-known that Richard's heart easily boiled with rage—he was capable of vehement emotions. In contrast, the idiom of the coward. "His heart beat like that of a rabbit," describes a heart racing in panic, or perhaps trembling like the leaf of an aspen.

The ancestors of the Germans of today used a very concrete approach to determine the courage of a person by measuring the size of their heart. In fact, they cut open the chests of their fallen enemies and if the heart was large, they knew that they had conquered a courageous opponent. However, a small heart that still twitched and trembled revealed itself to be the heart of a coward. In the figurative sense, one takes a similar approach today when one speaks on the one hand of a big-hearted person and on the other hand of those who are faint hearted and fickle-hearted. It is no coincidence that the U.S. Army medal for wounds in battle is the Purple Heart, while the red-purple color emphasizes the aspect of combative courage even further. Such heroes have offered their heart's blood as a sacrifice for their country. A person who fights with such fervor—who values his country before his own life—must obviously love his country from the depths of his heart.

The heart is not just an excellent barometer of emotion (from the Latin *emovere* meaning to move out). To emote is to send out feelings from the heart—the source from whence they are emerging. When, for whatever reason, one does not let the emotions out and suppresses them instead, they become blocked up in the heart; several idioms of language express this condition. Also, it is there that these repressed feelings cause trouble. They can put the heart under pressure and even disturb its rhythm and function. "I am never resentful, even if my heart should break," (Heinrich Heine). Shakespeare gives the same suggestion for therapy: "Give words to your pain: grief that does not speak presses the burdened heart until it breaks."

The wisdom of language very clearly establishes a relationship between the pressure on the heart and the pressure in life, as well as the heart's beating along with the rhythm of life. When the heart *misses a beat, gallops, beats irregularly,* or *races,* idioms of language indicate an emotional mood that has a very close correlation to the respective medical situation. A *galloping* or *racing* heart apparently belongs to a person who feels hunted, while a *constricted* heart indicates someone who is narrow-minded, and an *expansive* heart represents a person who is broad-minded.

Furthermore, it is conspicuous that language, and dialect in particular, has its own pathoanatomy through both lexical meaning and the onomatopoeic value of the words. One feels almost tempted to see dialect as an art form of the spoken word—in an analogous way to pop art. Expressions such as "only a hard heart can break," "burning heart," and "heartache" reveal a deep knowledge about the psychosomatic correlations within our center. A European adage expresses the common sentiment that "A sick heart lives within a person who is torn." Those with a *heart-rending* experience cannot process their feelings in an emotionally appropriate way and they will eventually experience their hearts being physically torn apart in a myocardial infarction. Before the attack (in the heart) occurs, one may have felt *shooting pains to the heart.* The heart may already be emotionally broken within, even before the patient has an opportunity to draw the necessary parallels to life. A *twitching heart* may indicate that one has endured too much trauma, so that the heart attack announces itself before it actually occurs—not at all hitting like the proverbial bolt out of the blue. Long before it happens, the heart must have been *cramped and depressed* within the body. It will have pounded often enough, probably insisting on its right to do its work in peace and not to be disturbed by all of the repressed emotions. A person who cannot listen to the emotions of her heart must eventually feel these physical warnings.

Also, whenever a person lets her heart (and her life) become difficult, or be made difficult, the heart will at some point lie in her chest as if it were a stone—perhaps even heavy, hard, and dead. In contrast, those who at least occasionally experience the idiomatic "weight off my chest" or even the proverbial "millstone has dropped from around my neck" have listened to the heart's emotional complaints now and then, and these more fortunate people take them seriously and so will have easier experiences. Their chests will feel freer and they will have "more room to breathe."

Outpourings of the heart in the figurative sense are important for relieving the burdened or overstrained heart. Whatever one does not permit to flow out remains inside and creates pressure. This is why it is healthy to let an overflowing heart speak. However, anyone who keeps her feelings to herself will suffer as a result. Whatever feelings do not empty from the heart in the figurative sense may build up over a long period of time and ultimately this energy may pour into the heart sac as a medical manifestation, such as a cardiac effusion. In German there is an old saying that this cardiac edema has its source in the "piss of the heart worm." Consequently, the old folk medicine takes this *gnawing heart worm* very seriously and the adage goes that when the worm has gnawed through the blood vessel, the person will die. Whether it is a worm or it is ambition that gnaws at the heart, the picture (of the heart being *eaten away* by such things as the worm of ambition) says a great deal about a situation that is threatening physical health. Who could be angry with such a *tortured* heart when it moves within the chest and screams in pain for help?

The heart cannot expect much help during our modern times since, at best, drugs will fight its pain while its cries for help remain ignored. However, even more serious consideration would probably not help much. Since our culture almost never speaks the language of the heart, hardly anyone understands it anymore.

In his essay "The Metaphor of the Heart in Literature." Horst Rüdiger unintentionally presented a very clear description of the situation: "Modern language and time have repressed the matters of the heart relating to the shy boarding-school daughter to favor the heart failure of the apparently robust manager. Instead of the heart withering away, heart death has settled into our society." In any case, both the shy boarding-school daughter and the apparently robust manager have one thing in common. They make a secret of their hearts, not letting them express their need to have what they respectively deserve. We will encounter both of these types of people later when we devote some time to the subject of blood pressure.

Folk medicine has always seen heart disorders as being of a higher calling, and usually considered their origins to be supernatural. A person afflicted at his center could not be considered an insignificant, harmless matter. This explains frequent attempts to heal heart problems with supernatural remedies. Demons were exorcised, lured out, and prayed out. This may seem primitive, but today we attempt to calm the stress demons with beta blockers and we fight the ghostly pressure to excel by exchanging the exhausted (heart) pump for a new one. We may very well consider those earlier attempts at therapy with a humility in our heart. Old folk medicine considered the heart to be a diversion for demons, noting that witches, vampires, and demons prefer to attack the heart and the blood—particularly the blood of the heart.

After all, folk medicine has known for several centuries what orthodox medicine is only now confirming scientifically in wide-scale studies: loneliness breaks the heart and a heart-disease patient is love-sick. There was a traditional remedy that many of our ancestors used to treat the pangs of love and emotional despondency (symptoms which we would refer to as depression today) and this was to make a sacrifice: a representative image, picture, or figurine of the heart, fashioned from whatever precious materials as the patient could afford. The affected person offered this precious heart (symbolizing his own) to God, Christ, or the Virgin Mary. He would certainly have been healed if he performed this ritual wholeheartedly. To give one's heart and open up to God's Creation has remained the most reliable therapy for every form of depression and disorder of the heart. The ancients knew very well that the heart should be considered either a *temple of God* (unity) or a *workshop of the devil* (polarity or divided state of being). In the first case, its owner was certain of salvation, and in the second case discord and despair were inevitable. Countless devotional pictures, with either God or a demon at the center, suggest this viewpoint. Even today we say that miserliness and greed *possess* a person's heart. The first of these vices makes the heart tight while the second puts it under pressure, both making it sick.

When one summarizes this study of the language of the heart, it is obvious that everything that constricts the heart, resulting in its hardening, leads to disease while everything that opens and widens the heart, contributing to its relief and liveliness, ultimately aims in the direction of love. One can differentiate even further on the basis of our idiomatic vocabulary. Whatever leads into the direction of a general opening up to life and to God has *healthy* (if not *wondrous)* effects. Once again, love takes on a narrower perspective if it is turned into something more individual, where it relates to just one specific person and thereby excludes all others. Therefore, such love might hurt accordingly and might also promote heart symptoms of the unpleasantly tight sort. The desire to "take someone into your heart" only to imprison and isolate him relates very closely to the closing or hardening of the heart. If your heart becomes *attached* to someone, you become tied to each other in the direct emotional sense of the word. If you *set your heart* on someone, you become stuck and cling to this person. Characteristically enough, one *joins* in a *matrimonial bond,* to which Goethe says, "Love is something idealistic, marriage is something realistic, and one can never mistake the idealistic for the realistic without being punished for doing so." The extreme of this path is the heart poisoned by jealousy, pretending to love passionately, yet eagerly searching for something that creates suffering.

In the impulses of the constricted heart as comprehended by language, one may also hear the exhortation to open oneself or open the heart. The heart pounding on the chest wall makes this perfectly clear. It acts as though it were a person pounding at a door; it expects and hopes to have the door answered. The scream uttered out of excess pressure is a plea for relief. Someone who feels painfully rock-hard is longing for tender gentleness. Depression and oppression call for something heartwarming. When the heart becomes cramped within the body, it begs for relaxation. If a person's chest is so tight up to his throat that she can hardly breathe, she apparently longs to release the bonds that tie her. The painfully contracted heart would feel great pleasure to stretch freely and take up space without pushing up against narrow boundaries. No matter what it is that is cramped, our idioms naturally classify it as depressed, sick, and sad. "A sad heart bums itself; it starves and dies of thirst" (Schi-King). In contrast, a wide, open heart appears to be the guarantee for vitality, health, heartiness, and a merciful attitude. Without a doubt, its perspective is one of unity, while the constricted, hard heart is one that breaks due to despair. When the heart *breaks,* all schools of medicine recognize this as a proverbial image of the most certain sign of approaching death.

    The fairy tales of various nations make up a treasure chest for our dictionary of the language of the heart. They know a great deal about the secrets of our center, as they have arisen from the oldest forms of human wisdom. The heart appears explicitly in some titles, as in the tale of the "Man without a Heart" (Bechstein) and "The Cold Heart" (Hauff). While in "The Frog Prince" (Brothers Grimm) for example, the faithful Henry had to have three iron bands put around his heart so that it would not burst because of his sadness about the prince. This suggests danger to the heart from clinging too loyally for too long; loyalty is at home in the heart—together with love and courage. At this point, we will take leave of the fairy tales and the wisdom of the proverbs and familiar quotations. However, colloquial language will continue to accompany us and will become an irreplaceable tool. It has an abundance of revealing information yet to give to us.

7.

The Heart and Love

Discourse about the heart leads quickly to the topic of love. All previous quotes from the Bible, from colloquial language, from fairy tales, and from proverbs point in this direction. Just as the heart's place is at the center of the body, love is a central requirement for life. Everything appears to point to love. Every individual ultimately wants to feel loved, more than anything else, but the paths and attempts at achieving this goal are extremely multitudinous and often quite diverse. They range from good behavior to external efforts, such as wearing attractive clothing and makeup, or attempts to earn recognition through outstanding achievement (as through the adulation of fame), and the desire of politicians to become so convincing and charismatic that everyone will vote for them. One recognizes the longing to be more lovable from behind the bloody procedures of cosmetic surgery and even many dictators—through the most brutal coercive measures—reveal their desire to have an entire population love them, without exception.

The attempt to force love through its opposites—war and violence—is as old as history and is always destined to fail. This is a classical allopathic approach. The homeopathic approach—gaining love through love—is incomparably more effective. Despite such an apparently promising starting point, one usually has a hard time with love, as did our ancestors. Christianity declares itself to be the religion of love, yet it has become the perfect example of how easy it is to practice the exact opposite when one attempts to force love. One only has to recall all the hatred and bloodshed associated with the witch trials of the Inquisition, or the horror of the Crusades against the Muslims, the Cathari, and the Templars. In the name of Christ, entire peoples have been massacred—from the American Indians, the Incas, and the Aztecs of the past to the crimes still perpetrated today against the remaining Indians of Latin America. Christian history is full of such aberrations, but personal histories usually display their fair share as well, and everybody has certainly experienced how easily love can turn into hatred. This polarity-changing process not only affects Christianity and to be fair to religion one must first look beneath the surface of this phenomenon—both in the realm of religion as well as with respect to ourselves. First we must set aside the drastic outer manifestations of history and then we must look to the depths of motivation and the sources of religion (Christ's own words being an example).

In view of the shocking atrocities that have already taken place in the name of love and religion, one might assume that this has always been a matter of error. Most people prefer to interpret things this way, especially in the area of personal relationships. One usually assumes that the wrong person merely happened to be the object to whom one gave one's heart. Although it is only human to blame the unwilling object of our love for our failure, this hardly helps. Even brief reflection reveals that the people over whom we choose to become obsessive are practically arbitrary. There is hardly anything on this earth that has not already been both loved and hated. One may love one's partner and one's cat, one's homeland, the earth, motorcycling, roast pork on Sundays, wind surfing, peace, disco, snowball fights, sunsets at the ocean, and a beer after work. There is nothing that we cannot love. Only our own notions—which change at a relatively fast pace—stand in the way of such an understanding. It may be difficult to imagine that the Romans loved their cruel gladiator fights, while today many people love boxing or car racing. Others prefer the circus, where the acrobats and aerial artists endanger their lives in order to entertain the audience. It is precisely this thrill of danger that the spectators love. Without any doubt, everything one detests today was loved at some other time. In addition, everything that is loved today was once loathed. Fashion demonstrates how quickly and arbitrarily this change can occur. In any case, this reasoning does not move us any further forward since apparently everything, without exception, can be loved or hated to the same degree.

From the object of love let us move now to its place of origin, and so back to ourselves. All previous studies have shown that the heart is the organ and the home of love. As the center of the circulatory system and strongest rhythmic organ, it regulates the vital rhythm and the feeling within the center of one's life. The heart is our center. From an energy viewpoint as well: *Anahata,* the corresponding chakra or energy center, is what Eastern traditions consider to be the middle of the seven large energy vortices of the body. Also, just as everything in life revolves around love, everything on the energy level revolves around the heart center. On the functional level, the heart has the assignment of keeping the life energy (symbolized in the blood) flowing, and the same principle functions on the emotional level, where it is love that keeps us flowing and therefore alive.

A precise look at the functioning of the heart reveals many parallels to what we have already gathered from language. This relates to the act of taking something in and letting it continue to flow, to giving vital impulses. The heart must continually *open up* to the incoming blood—it must completely *accept it* and *let it in;* in a similar way that we open our hearts lovingly and let in what we love. On the other hand, a serious difference between the heart and the expression of love becomes clear at this. The heart accepts all the blood that comes to it—without exception! It does not discriminate between individual blood cells or certain components of the blood. Also, it does not hold on to anything! On the contrary, it immediately releases everything it has just accepted so that it can continue to flow—at least, as long as it remains healthy. If it becomes ill, it begins to hold back an increasingly large portion of the blood (called residual blood). Openness, expansiveness, and flow are the dominant symbols of the physical heart, while opposite tendencies naturally come into play whenever one tends to impede the object of love from continuing to flow (in order to keep it for oneself). In addition, such attempts again brings the opposite pole much closer than is appropriate.

Expansiveness and openness are qualities belonging to the physically healthy and loving heart, while withdrawing, narrowing, and fear are the opposite. Wherever health and love are lacking, one will meet the opposite pole—fear. Hate (mentioned earlier as the shadow counterpart of love) also has its roots on this polarity.

An understanding of the development of the heart can even take us one step further. During the first nine months of life—the time in the womb—the heart works as a single chamber with just one circulatory system. The embryo still lives in clear proximity to the unity of Paradise. One finally reaches the divided world of polarity with birth and with the first breath of air. From that moment on, everything has its opposite and meaning is established through this polarity. For newborns, the polarity begins with the inhalation and exhalation of the breath, a process that will accompany them for as long as they live. Indeed, inhalation is just as dependent on exhalation as the reverse. The heart, more closely connected to the Unity than the lungs, has been beating since the formation of the fetus. A newborn usually experiences this transition from the Unity into this divided world with conflicting feelings and quite often with despair. Both lungs unfurl through the first breath, causing the reflexive closing of the heart septum and thereby the division of the heart into two parts. From this point on, doctors speak of the left heart and the right heart. From this moment there are two circulations in the body—the large (systemic) circulation and the lesser (pulmonary) circulation.

Now the opposite poles are not only separated on the physical level but have also become separated on the emotional level—even if they are frequently quite close to one another. They are so close that in the twinkling of an eye, fondness can turn into antipathy and love can ferment into hate. However, once again the body has little difficulty in dealing with these polarities. It attaches the same importance to both sides and is not judgmental. The right heart receives just as much blood as the left heart. We prefer the one more pleasant side of reality. We hope that the other side will disappear if we ignore it. However, as we already know, this is impossible. It will merely dive into the shadow to rise up again as soon as its time has come. Also, it usually comes more quickly but in any case less pleasantly than one would like. A persistently repressed side of reality will attract attention with equal pressure (by becoming a symptom, for example). This may also serve to explain why the Christian church, with all its passionate aspiration to love, has had to express so much hatred. It also illustrates why relationships that began in ardent love can end in such cold hatred.

In summary, from birth—or, viewed mythologically, from Adam's and Eve's expulsion from Paradise—we inhabit a world of opposites that tends to bring both sides to light eventually. Therefore, as we emphasize one side and suppress the other, the suppressed aspect will certainly try to emerge from the underground. However, the heart is an organ that can mediate, a fact evident in its symbol (two curves strive towards one middle) as well as its position in the center of the body between the two poles. Therefore, the heart becomes our gateway from polarity into unity. When one opens the heart, one may find heaven (unity) on earth. This permits us to remove the earthly bonds that bind the individual to the opposites for a time (for example, when one is in love) or forever (the state of illumination or, in Christian terms, the state of eternal life). As the core, the heart is also a symbol of this possibility since every center offers the opportunity of reaching another, deeper level. And so it is the Buddhist goal to reach the center of the wheel of reincarnation in order to escape the eternal cycle of births in polarity.

The Heart and Love

One may further determine that everything is lovable at a basic level. It is always just a question of relative values. Once more, the heart presents a perspective of the goal of all development. It does not judge, it opens itself for everything and everyone. Finally, observation of the heart and its functions also confirms a definition of love that language has already revealed. To love means to open up and to let something in—completely unfettered from all of the many objects of love. Love always correlates with the idea of uniting. This presumes that one opens one's own borders and expands oneself

Sexuality, as the coarsest level of love (because it is physical), confirms this definition for us. Mainly involving body orifices, the characteristic purpose of sex is to penetrate as deeply as possible into another person—to create an ultimate unity during orgasm. The precondition for this deep merging is in turn to open to each other and to expand. Then during orgasm, it is possible to cross the boundaries of the polarity for a brief moment and to experience a feeling of unity. This state of oneness with everything is the typical feeling for a person who dwells in the center—in the heart.

The definition of love (as an opening and expansion) in turn exposes hatred on the opposite pole (as a closing and becoming constricted). However, narrowness is fear. A confidently open person will consequently be big-hearted and generally ready to love, while a closed, tense person is, by way of contrast, narrow-minded and fearful—tending to be more willing to hate. Physics gives us an analogy for this in its definition of the process of warming. In this process, an expansion of the molecular pattern takes place through the increased mobility of the individual molecules. Therefore, the warmer a body is, the further its molecules move apart, while the colder a body is, the closer the molecules draw together. Warmth is clearly also the quality that we connect with love. This is why we also speak of *warm*-hearted people, *hot* love, and *burning* hearts. Coldness also relates to fear, as we can see in expressions such as "a chill down my back" and "I got cold feet." A cold heart belongs to a hateful face and it certainly does not belong to a warmhearted person. Cold-blooded behavior is calculating; never coming from a warm heart but from a cold mind—principally ruled more by fear than by love.

All this leads to understanding of the paradox; all people essentially strive for the same prize—namely love—and yet the world is rather loveless. The pleasant thing about love is actively opening up and letting the other person in while, in contrast, a passive waiting for love brings little satisfaction or only disappointment. Opening up inner boundaries, expanding the heart, and giving the heart to someone else are all active actions that challenge the individual and her barriers. Only if one voluntarily gives up these limitations and boundaries (that secure the ego and isolate at the same time) is it possible to unite with the other person and gain that warm feeling that one calls love and enjoys so much. This emotion is increasingly overwhelming the more we open up and the more of the world we let in.

Let us consider fear in more detail as the opposite pole of love. Although everybody has an enormous need for love, one has an even greater fear of opening one's boundaries. This starts with the very mundane borders of our garden fences and the borders surrounding our countries. Everything outside of us that is foreign creates fear and it is against our natural instincts to want to welcome it. It could disturb one's state of security or even challenge the ego in many different ways. All the foreigners who want to enter a country could disturb it or might even want to participate in the wealth of one's country and so one closes the boundaries or does not open up at all or, even better, one pretends to open the boundaries without actually doing so. This brings us precisely back to the situation a person finds herself in—she does not truly open up because she has too much fear of what she might find on the outside. At best, she behaves in a simulation of openness, and she waits for love. Although other people might accept this game and not be equally distracted by their own fearful waiting, this would not help us. If being adored is the solution to a happy life, all the movie and pop stars would be the happiest people in the world and yet precisely the opposite appears to be the case, wherein a large fraction of all celebrities seem to have been searching for love for their entire lives.

Each person can only take the decisive step of opening up their own boundaries for their own sakes and one can only be happy if one really does so. Simply tearing down the fence that the ego has built against the rest of the world already conveys this unique feeling of expansion, warmth, and happiness. This fence disappears in a state of love; it feels so indescribably unrestrained and boundless that anyone who has once experienced this state longs to return to it. Within it, one practically lives outside of time and space, one can live on love and air alone, one exists from within one's own center. This consciousness feels so *heavenly* because unity is so close. It is one of the few precious moments in life that is uncritical and unconditional, a moment outside of the polarity or between the poles—in the center of the heart.

The Unity evades our polarized perception (completely built on contrariness and comparison) and it also eludes description through language, since language imperatively depends upon the comparative and boundary-setting possibilities of the polarity. However, one may gain an impression of this from two people who share this feeling of merging for a moment. Orgasm is such an opportunity. Both of the lovers have come as close as possible to one another and they have found a mutual rhythm of movement, and resonate in harmony. For this moment they share the same wavelength, and so orgasm—the experience of unity—is possible.

Resonance is an essential experience of love and a prerequisite for experiencing unity. When they resonate with each other, both of the lovers open themselves up to another level that would have remained closed to them as individual beings. They illustrate the wise old saying, "the whole is more than the sum of its parts." One may utterly understand the process of falling in love as entering a state of resonance. Two people open up to one another, find their mutual rhythm, and connect with each other on a higher level. The expression "falling in love" makes this correlation very clear. From one moment to the next, the two appear to fall into this special state of resonance.

This phenomenon spans completely different fields. For example, the military knows that marching in step is much easier to manage than each soldier choosing his own rhythm. The resonance within such a troop is also the reason for its great strength. Such vibrations can even cause great bridges to collapse. A more appropriate example for our context comes from medical science. If two isolated heart cells come into proximity—each pulsing in completely different rhythms—their rhythms will adjust to each other even before they touch. In pictorial terms, they fall into resonance. Were they not individual cells but whole heart organs, one might say that they "fell in love." Our language helps us even further in expressing this phenomenon in the everyday interpersonal area. If one feels a sympathetic connection to someone, a mysterious closeness exists—an inexplicable and invisible link. One is open for this person or receptive to him or her. If the transmitter and receiver have the same frequency, one is on the same "wavelength" and *unison* prevails, one is in resonance with the other. Anyone who has experienced this knows that it is not an intellectual phenomenon since it can also take place between two people who do not even speak the same language. The secret lies much deeper, namely in the heart. These hearts resonate on the same level and, as the adage goes, "The two of them are tuned-in to each other."

This perspective illuminates a variety of love phenomena—for example why opposites attract. When two completely different people succeed in opening to each other and letting their hearts unite, they have managed to span a wide gulf. This requires an enormous opening, and opening ourselves is the most pleasant feeling that we know. In proportion to the difference between their original rhythms the shared rhythm is new and more overwhelming, connecting, and binding. Love that successfully goes this far is beyond doubt, and only great, unconditional love can build such a bridge. The love between children and their animals is often of this form, but the example of Romeo and Juliet is as typical as it is famous.

There is an explanation for the belief that love has the power to change a person drastically. It is quite possible that the new mutual level of resonance is a good distance away from an individual's old level. In "love at first sight," one utterly and unexpectedly falls into a new level of resonance, which practically transforms its subject from one moment to the next. One is *madly* in love.

On this basis, we can better understand the apparently contradictory "opposites attract," and "birds of a feather flock together." People are not always open enough to bridge wide gulfs. In this case, it is naturally good to find someone who is similar or has nearly the same type of nature. The small leap to emotional resonance is possible—at least one is no longer alone. Loneliness is the least resonant and therefore most unpleasant condition possible. There is definitely a reason for solitary confinement also being called isolation torture. For human beings, who are social creatures, this is most certainly one of the crudest punishments. The loneliness of the heart is one of the most dangerous risk factors that medical studies have been able to determine to date. However, voluntary solitude bears opportunity—such as during spiritual exercises. When the aloneness becomes an all-oneness, a person will resonate in complete harmony with himself and he automatically enters into a state of unison with everyone and everything else.

This is the state of self-realization that the East calls illumination and Christian culture considers to be eternal life. It is no coincidence that one finds this state of consciousness at that point. If unity requires resonance, illumination must naturally relate to resonance. A person who has achieved self-realization feels herself to be one with all other people and creatures and so she feels utterly unified with all of creation—at any rate, such is the description given by the mystics. This means that such a person resonates in unison with everything and is also in harmony with everything. Today, modem physics teaches us that everything is vibration and connected with everything else. This may impart to us an intuition that love (the only thing that allows us to feel this bond) represents a basic force of creation that is at least equal to destruction—that other basic force.

The experience of being connected to everything corresponds to the all-embracing unconditional love that one also calls divine love and it correctly seems to be quite distant, not to mention that it appears in heaven. In the same way, one imagines God's love to be boundless and so one naturally expects God to include everybody in His love and to exclude nobody. It is therefore not sensible when one feels tempted to say, "God does not love me anymore; He has forsaken me in favor of my neighbor." For God, unconditional and boundless openness simply cannot be renounced.

In contrast, people tend to set conditions and therefore set boundaries and thus one tends to separate oneself from others. The ego acts this way because of fear. The ego exists entirely because of the existence of boundaries, which makes this completely justified. It wants to be special and definitely wants to avoid being submerged into the boundless sea of unity. Its entire energy is focused on setting boundaries for itself and so dramatizing itself One might even describe its actual nature as one of creating boundaries and ambition is the best vehicle for realizing this goal. Therefore, every form of love threatens the survival of the ego, as love endangers the fences that the ego has struggled to build. However, all-encompassing love is the end of all boundaries and safeguards—it represents the death of the ego.

It is understandable, then, that the ego will attempt to prevent love and will even try to obstruct the steps leading to love with panic-stricken fear—that is why a person with a very strong ego cannot fall in love very easily and even if they do so, it is unlikely to be an eternal love. Also, if the experience of love should happen, it would be difficult for the person to make the necessary sacrifices. He would find it difficult to risk being disinherited, or to forgo a career, or even to give up a personally advantageous relationship. The ego is also very calculating in this respect and

The Heart and Love

so, when concerned with its own survival, several arguments will always seem to surface that denigrate one's great love—or at least attempt to dismantle it piece by piece. The methods are very familiar; the ego will simply make a few seemingly reasonable demands or request concrete evidence of this love. However, once a person has fallen in love, a very powerful ego is needed to close the wide-open gates of the heart. In such a state of love, the ever-powerful ego is more or less unimportant. It is easy to recognize this state because the affected person is not the least bit insecure about his love, ignoring arguments that may even be extremely reasonable and sensible. In its concern for its own existence, the ego does not care about the possible consequence that it might destroy a person's chance for happiness with its antics.

Since the ego exists through its defined boundaries, it is the opposite pole of self-realization and the greatest enemy of love. This is why the Bible also refers to it as Satan. It strives to establish sharp differences everywhere—separation, division, schisms, and duality. For this reason, the Bible constantly warns us not to permit Satan into our hearts. If the ego lakes command at this single point of connection to unity, then eternal life is a great distance away and any form of love can only be achieved with great difficulty. Only with an open heart may one realize divinity in other people and only with an open and pure heart is one capable of recognizing God in everything.

The Christian religion—as well as nearly every other religion—ultimately sets these high standards for mankind. The Native-American chief Dan George formulated this credo in particularly uncompromising terms, "The human being must love the entire Creation, or he will love nothing in it." Christ lived and preached such divine boundless love, a form of love that knows no differences, relating to one's neighbor in exactly the same way as it does to oneself, and even expressly includes one's enemies. This love desires to become one with everything, its objective being redemption from the ego (and therefore from Satan). Yet Christians have often taken another path, one that is apparently even more demanding. They have turned the sentence "Love your neighbor as yourself" into "Love your neighbor more than anything else." This guide for behavior has already taken these believers a good distance away from themselves. Although Christ's commandment was clearly directed towards the individual, this alternate version leaves the door wide open for the creation of the shadow. Since Christians were unable to love themselves, which would mean having to accept themselves with all their weaknesses, naturally they could not love their neighbors. When a person is not truly open with herself, it is much more difficult to open up to others and she may at best pretend that she is open. In addition, this is the same way that Christian churches became a community of people who only act as though they were open to others. It is hard to conceive of a better prerequisite for the growth of the shadow and so it has not taken long for the forceful appearance of many contradictions to the much sworn and oft quoted love. Naturally, it was difficult for individual believers to fulfill Christ's commandment and practice a love that overcomes all boundaries when their own church was doing everything it could to set boundaries and to achieve power. Therefore, the Church threw its lot in with the main opponent of all-encompassing love—namely the ego, or Satan, as the Bible would say.

Christians have virtually ignored Christ's second central statement on this topic, or else they have transformed it into its opposite. In the Church's own politics, the word *destroy* has apparently replaced *love* in the sentence "love your enemies." In this respect, many believers have followed this easier path. However, the original sentence reflects enormous potential. Enemies represent a concentrated version of everything that one rejects and shuts out in the mind. Enemies embody the projection of whatever one cannot stand within oneself. If only we could succeed in opening ourselves to precisely all of this, if only we could allow it into our heart instead of so vehemently denying it, then we would find we had reached the goal of our development and were in a state of divine love. Instead, our usual response is to attempt to destroy these enemies. Yet, as I have already pointed out, this is impossible since whatever a person tries to eradicate will eventually end up in another location or—after all the effort spent in being rid of it—it will appear in one's own shadow.

There is an interesting association here with those special, inner enemies—our symptoms, which accompany us along the course of life for long stretches. Most people regard symptoms as enemies that they would rather eliminate. If one could succeed in learning to love these enemies in accordance with the Christian commandments (that would mean opening one's heart and accepting the symptoms) one would realize that they contain an immense potential for inner development. In their symbolic language, these symptoms explain to us which problems they represent and which aspects of them we reject. If the patient could succeed in reintegrating this basic principle that he has rejected, he would be a bit closer to wholeness and he would have traveled the road of development a good deal further. All this is yet another reason to turn with an attitude of unbiased openness and love to one's symptoms.

Part 2

I.
The Language of the Heart

1.

The Heart's Structure and How It Works

Even the form and the function of a heart that is healthy and working normally provides an abundance of information about its significance and its purpose in both a concrete and a figurative sense. Again, it is language that offers us valuable assistance in its psychosomatic duality.

From the beginning of modern times, images from the realm of poetry and nature have described the heart and its work, one such image being that of an unfolding rose. With the triumphant advance of mechanistic thinking, the view of the heart has become increasingly technological—as a pump, subject to the newly discovered laws of hydraulics. In the following paragraphs, when we also use image and metaphor to open access into the world of the heart, it is important to make it clear from the outset that the truth lies somewhere between all of these metaphorical descriptions. The heart naturally has, when it lovingly opens itself, a similar relationship to a tender, unfolding, or budding rose. When one speaks of a person who is blossoming one is referring to his heart in particular. The analogy with the rose goes even further since the rose is the ultimate queen of flowers, while the heart is the queen or king of the organs. The heart is neither feminine nor masculine, which reveals the limitations of such assignments. Between these two polarities, it beats at the center. Its special position and the clear relationship to the central point also stands out in this respect. A similar situation is only true for the brain, although less emphatically.

On the other hand, one can also naturally compare the heart to the engine of an automobile, since the heart is the center of the energy supply and it keeps the entire human machine running. To do even more Justice to the heart, one may use the picture of the two-stroke engine that does its tactful work between drawing in and expelling its gases. However the analogy ends here; the heart beats with its special rhythm and does not use cylinders. The relationship of rhythm and stroke is similar to that of life and death. In addition, it would certainly be a miraculous engine if it could grow along with the growth of a car and even continue to work while it grows. Imagine a car that grows and adapts through time with a growing family. Later, when the family becomes smaller again, this wondrous car would shrink and adapt itself to the new circumstances. It would be the perfect procession of metamorphosis from baby carriage, to tricycle, to bicycle, to the first four-wheeler, at its best a sports car, then to a station wagon, and finally back to a sedan.

The heart leads us far beyond technology's limitations and well into the world of wonders (as do all of our organs). One must admit that the heart is far and away beyond the most sophisticated man-made technology and its associated principles. Even within the common mechanistic picture of the world, the heart far outperforms the potential of today's technology as it executes approximately one hundred thousand beats per day, circulates nearly three thousand gallons of blood (the load of a normal tank truck), and performs these duties—uninterrupted—for approximately seventy years without any explicit maintenance or repair. The coronary vessels expand and stretch one-hundred-thousand times a day during the process of the heart's action. Is there any technological device that could stand up to such treatment for seventy years or more? Such information may be quite interesting for our intellectual understanding, but it also instills a certain reverence for the heart and its work. Also, such reverence is essential in order to later understand the problems of the heart and—above all—to accept them.

Keeping in mind the limitations of technical analogies, we can compare the heart's work to a pump system in the center of a plumbing network. I have previously mentioned Harvey and his analogy to the solar system, so let us now think of the heart as the center of a hydraulic circulatory system with two valves. In this picture, the heart is a high-performance pump that presses the water outward into the pipes, supplying as much pressure as needed in order for sufficient water to be available anywhere in the pipe system. No matter how high the water faucets might be above the pumping station—whether on the fourteenth floor of a skyscraper, or far up in the head of the physical body—the pump in the heart of the city, or the body, must provide the city, or body, with adequate pressure. The organs and tissues of the organism correspond to the customers of the water company. As long as the pump works, it guarantees the necessary pressure to the water supply. However, if the central pump stops working, the pressure in the entire pipe would quickly drop. The result would be that the households, or the organs, could no longer receive their supply.

However, this is where the comparison breaks down since the failure of a municipal water system is merely unpleasant while, to a human, any type of circulatory standstill very quickly becomes life-threatening. After just five seconds, the brain (the highest-positioned household) already exhibits the first functional disorders. After ten seconds, the threatening situation becomes evident by the onset of unconsciousness—probably for the purpose of maintaining some of the vital fluids by shifting them downwards. After about eight minutes, the brain (household) usually suffers irreparable damage. Even if the pump were to go back into action (for example by direct heart massage) it would be too late for the central control station. It could no longer fulfill its function of maintaining order in the metaphorical city (of the human body). In order to prevent such catastrophes, various security measures protect the pumping center.

One of these security measures consists of a variety of pump-installed electronic alarm systems (networks of nerves). Another is that the heart pump itself is the initial recipient of its own energy output. It is the first to receive the vital fluids that leave its left ventricle through the coronary vessels. These coronaries form a garland around the heart, in the truest sense of the word, and they provide all of the heart cells with fresh energy. If there is an abrupt interruption in this supply (such as the constriction of angina pectoris) then intense pain—another of the organism's warning systems—occurs immediately. If the supply completely shuts off (as in a heart attack) unimaginable pain is adequate to signal the alarm.

The municipal water pipes correspond metaphorically to the arteries, which transport the fresh blood to the organs and tissues. A municipal sewage and waste system corresponds to the veins that return used blood to the heart. The metaphor falters at this point since the cardiopulmonary system implements perfect recycling (which remains an unfulfilled dream for the engineers of any waterworks).

We have considered the heart's function as it relates to the surrounding organs and so let us now focus on the heart alone. It weighs between three hundred and five hundred grams and its size is roughly that of a person's clenched fist. It is a hollow muscle located approximately in the middle of the chest—shifted a bit to the left (the feminine or emotional side of the body). The heart beats on an average of seventy times per minute—more than four thousand beats in an hour. This represents about three billion heartbeats in seventy years of human life.

The simple schematic sketch shown in Illustration 1 portrays the path that the blood takes through the heart. The blood arrives from the lungs—laden with fresh oxygen energy and relieved of carbon dioxide wastes—and reaches the left atrium. The heart stretches and expands in its relaxation phases (diastole) while the blood flows out of the atrium into the ventricle—whereby

Heart-Aches

the mitral valve[6] swings open like a double door and offers no resistance to the flow of blood. Next, the tension phase follows (systole) as the increasing pressure pushes back both cusps of the mitral valve and the valve's double doors slam together, whereby they form a barrier in the middle position and no longer open up to the ventricle.

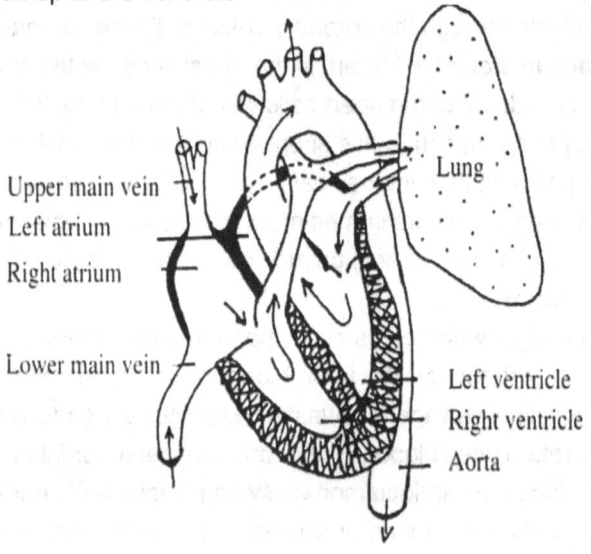

Illustration 1

At the exit of the left heart ventricle to the aorta, there is also a valve set in the other direction. During the tension phase, the blood can stream out into the circulatory system, but not back into the now empty ventricle. The other side (right side) of the heart functions exactly the same way in principle. The blood flows through the aorta (the main artery) to the organs and tissues, then it streams back and returns through the upper and lower vena cava to the heart, namely into the right atrium. During the relaxation phase it flows into the right heart atrium and from there it passes through the tricuspid valve, corresponding to the left valve on the opposite atrium but which has an additional cusp. In the next tension phase, the right ventricle releases blood into the lungs where it re-oxygenates and returns to the left atrium.

In addition to the movement-energy, the heart also provides the blood with a clear direction. Therefore, it performs the equally important task of preventing the *river of life* from changing directions. Blood, which is often called the nectar of life—a symbol of vital energy, must only flow forward and the swinging double doors of the heart valves guarantee this. The division of the heart into a right and a left heart provides order; the septum separates the lesser (or pulmonary) circulatory system, which serves to regenerate the blood, from the general (or systemic) circulatory system, which guarantees the supply of energy to all the tissue and organs and thereby to all the living cells.

The division of the heart into two sections has a direct correspondence to life in our world of polarities, where everything has its two sides. This opposing nature is necessary for order. Therefore, the formation of the cardiac septum, which separates the heart chambers before birth, is a necessity for life in this world. Before the point of birth, the fetus is so close to the Unity that it has only one large heart ventricle and a single circulatory system. With the first breath, the actual entrance into polarity, both lobes of the lungs unfurl. Only then does the pulmonary circulatory system join together in its dual action. This in turn closes the large embryonic opening of the cardiac septum, which thereby divides the heart in the middle. Most newborns experience this abrupt change into the world of duality with some despair.

However, this occurrence in the physical body is essential. When the closing of the septum is aborted or does not fully complete, folk language calls the condition a hole in the heart while doctors refer to it as a cardiac defect. These afflicted newborns have not managed to take the symbolic step into the world of duality but have remained close to the Unity instead. However, this often leads to death on the physical level. If the infant—often with the help of modern surgery or medication—stays alive, these children have great difficulties incarnating themselves in the truest sense of the word. They turn blue from the exertion of every small physical effort. Surgery to seal shut the hole in the septum is the best way to help them. These desperate operations are an approach to forcing life by splitting the heart with great trauma and violation.

On the basis of its development, the heart has a relationship to both the unity of Paradise beyond this world and to conflicted human existence in this polarized world. Its symbolism brings both sides together in one sign (see Illustration 2). Beneath the two heart curves is a pit that allows the two halves to become one again. This basic polarity also finds expression through a normal heart function. In systole, the heart compresses itself to its maximum, becoming small and hard and closed in upon itself. The diastole that follows stretches and opens the heart up to its limits, and in the process it widens and prepares itself to accept everything (blood).

We have used a mechanical metaphor for the heart function and now we must also direct our attention to its control. In accordance with the heart as our center, the heart's rhythm regulates its work from within rather than from the outside. One might call it autonomous. However, the environment outside the heart can clearly influence its rhythm because the heart is not isolated and, in fact, it interacts very closely with all other body systems. Above all, the heart receives substantial influence from the brain stem. However, the actual pulse generator lies within the heart itself. Comparable to a transmitter, it sends its signals to all heart cells through the stimulus conducting system. These electrical impulses are the basis of the ECG (electrocardiogram), which can provide diagnostic information on the heart's conduction system. The sinoatrial node is the transmitter within the heart and is composed from unique tissue—half nerve and half muscle—that has developed from muscle cell tissue. Evidently, the heart has had to acquire its autonomy in the course of a long evolution. It is possible that this development occurred in parallel with the achievement of human autonomy—at a time when the human being reflected about himself as an individual being.

The Heart's Structure and How It Works

Even today when a person says "I," one points exactly to where the heart resides and beats its autonomous rhythm.

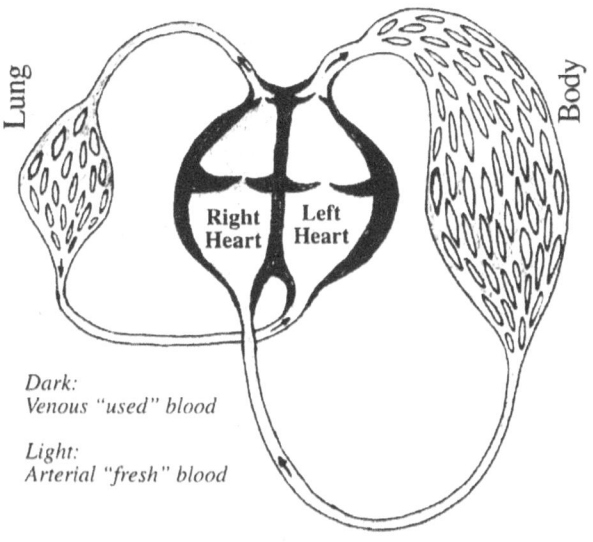

Dark:
Venous "used" blood

Light:
Arterial "fresh" blood

Illustration 2

On the other hand, the special pulse-generating cells of the sinoatrial node are not so unique, which reflects their origin very clearly. They distinguish themselves from the other cells of the conduction system only through their higher impulse frequency. If the sinoatrial node fails, the heart does not lack a pulse generator. Instead, the subordinate part of the conduction system, the so-called AV node (atrioventricular node) then sets the rate to a lower frequency—in accordance with its subordinate position. If this pulse center fails, then the heart cells themselves can still transmit their signal, but the frequency is too low for survival. In addition, many clashes for dominance will occur in that event. The hierarchy of the top of the genetic pulse-power pyramid is strictly organized and it has very little latitude on which to base its regulation of hereditary succession. As long as the appropriate power is in the appointed cells, everything is in rhythmic order. However, if the hierarchy collapses, then all of the cells begin to have a say and they will try to govern and the rhythm decays into chaos. Usually, the pulse from the seat of government, the sinoatrial node, is so strong that it easily drowns out all of the other voices from the realm of the heart and asserts itself. From the outset, the sinoatrial node overrides all possible competitors, so that its activity causes an electrical depolarization and the node cells lose power with every new beat. This means, however, that the top of the hierarchy must at no time become weaker because a revolution would be the immediate consequence. Any general weakening in the dominant position of the conduction tissue will create a danger of anarchy in the heart.

In a healthy normal state, the heart tissue is a perfect example of cooperative behavior, as all of the multitude individual cells pull together simultaneously. Closely considered, this may appear to be something of a wonder. A suitable metaphor would be a huge school of fish which, although it consists of myriad individuals, may react as a single being. This image is very appropriate, as the heart muscle cells even have a certain spindle-shaped similarity to the fish, but are more closely bundled.

This is an impressive example of resonance. Even down to the function of each of its individual cells, the heart exhibits the pattern of love. In the healthy heart, all of the cells are supporting one another, without exception. They are responsible for each other and receive impulses from their mutual center. They are open and accessible, willing to respond at any moment. Very tightly packed, they are close to each other and attach as much importance to each neighbor as to themselves. They interact through their pattern of vibration and are mutually connected, even though they may reside in very different areas of the heart. The strict synchronization of this pattern of vibration also corresponds to the rigid order in the physical pattern of the muscle parts, as they wind around the heart in various layers, and so form the heart's structure.

With its impulses, the heart controls our life rhythm in coordination with the influences it receives from the brain. The autonomic nervous system influences it, but the heart may also exert influence through it. Emotions that come from the center can

The Heart's Structure and How It Works

sweep along the entire organism; one example of this is letting ourselves become enraptured. According to the understanding of orthodox medicine, the physical basis for such a state of rapture lies in the nerve connections to the external environment, which are located in the heart's periphery. They connect through the so-called cardiac plexus with the other autonomous (related to the viscera) nerve centers and to the *top*. In Eastern medicine, the energy paths explain this connection—the *meridians* of the Chinese, the *Nadis* of the Indians, and the Hindu *chakras* of the energy body. According to the latest scientific research, one can even assume that the heart also influences the entire body through its management of hormones. In this context, the right atrium is the designated source of a substance that lowers blood pressure.

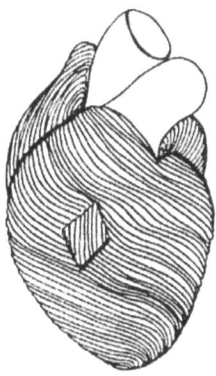

Illustration 3

It should also be mentioned that we can approach the heart (as suggested in many poetic metaphors) in another physiological respect as a sensory organ. Nerve paths are seldom one-way streets and so the heart receives just as much information from them as it transmits. The heart organ apparently adapts itself to a great variety of changing external circumstances. For example, it must provide the necessary additional energy for the movement of the limbs. However, to do so, it requires information that it receives about the extent of these movements. It has a sensory system for the circulatory process that also includes the ability to measure blood pressure. Very recently we have learned that the heart is even capable of registering temperature differences, such as the difference between the warmer blood of the lower body region, particularly in the liver, and the cooler blood of the upper half of the body.

The many capabilities and full potential of the heart have certainly not been explored fully in this abridged portrayal. However, the information presented here should form an adequate basis for our efforts to understand better the heart's physical expressions and its organic language.

2.

The Heart Out of Balance

Idioms, adages, and proverbs have always portrayed a big heart as standing for bravery and generosity, courage, and the ability to love. In one German dialect, "big-hearted" also refers to large breasts and actually indicates a woman who is courageous enough to express her femininity in an assertive manner. Expressions relating to small hearts are less common, but one may well assume that it represents the opposite pole. Expressions such as *fainthearted, weak-hearted, narrow-minded* (narrow-hearted), and *small hearted* (heartless) contrast with *big-hearted* and *magnanimous*. Finally, we consider the German idiom "hare's heart" which certainly refers to a small heart with a cowardly manifestation because of the hare's perpetual tendency to flee.

However, how does this relate to the concrete physical size of the heart? What is the significance of size? One rarely knows the size of one's own heart, since as long as there are no problems in this respect, there is no need to know. As any muscle does, the heart will also gain in size, weight, and strength to meet the demands placed upon it. In the case of a so-called cardiac enlargement, the muscle cells can double in number if exertion or excessive strain continues on a regular basis. Constantly raised blood pressure or regular high-performance training can cause this. Athletes who engage in endurance training at a high-performance level sometimes have such a cardiac enlargement and this is called *athletic heart*. To a certain point, athletic training is even beneficial for the cardiovascular system. However, when cardiac enlargement begins to cause problems it becomes like any other heart disease. As with any symptom, it stands for a shadow, a repressed problem that one has not consciously perceived and processed. In the case of pathological cardiac enlargement, with its tendency to decline into heart failure, this is naturally even more apparent.

As always, the symptom points to something that the patient did not previously recognize within himself and, therefore, does not consciously process. In this case, it shows the patient how large—as well as overstrained—the heart has already become, and that it has the tendency to continue to grow even further. In the figurative sense, the heart has really expanded—grown—beyond its limitations, and has become overtaxed. The affected person is not aware of her emotional heart size and her demands in this respect. She does not meet those demands in her life and so the theme sinks from consciousness into the shadow and demands attention in the body as a symptom.

In the field of sports, the high requirements on the heart (in the figurative sense) also become apparent in the arenas of Olympic ancient Greece. The athletes of that time had to be well-rounded men. It would have been unthinkable to equate the competing medal-seekers with mere high-performance machines. Baron Pierre de Coubertin (the founder of the modem Olympic Games in 1896) also supported the ancient Greek ideals, which have not withstood the materialism of the twentieth century. Today, the goal is to be the best, and participation hardly counts. The material aspects of Olympic Gold have completely outstripped the ideals that originated it. Winners and sponsors turn their gold into cash as quickly as possible and likewise physical cardiac enlargement has replaced the expansiveness of the heart.

The physical heart must now extend vicariously well beyond its own boundaries. In this case it becomes quite clear that the symbolic meaning of the symptom fits better into the emotional level. The expansion of the heart is emotionally pleasant and developmentally beneficial for the affected person and for his environment, however it demands much courage—even magnanimity and big-heartedness, according to folk idiom. In contrast, cardiac enlargement on the physical level is at best unpleasant and at worst life-threatening.

For athletes, cardiac enlargement usually is not a problem during their active years but, it often does become a problem at the close of a career. This, in turn, is easy to understand since as long as the athlete is active she works through her problem with persistence, and makes adjustments if necessary; she constantly strives to surpass herself and to break all limitations and records. So her theme is present in the training ritual that requires her to test herself every day and, even if she does not resolve this theme, she will work it through with much energy and vigor. When the athlete stops training, she could of course process this problem in the emotional sense by opening her heart to her family or by starting to live heartily in some other manner, thus growing beyond her emotional limitations. If she fails to reach this level, or to find an emotional substitute for her sport, she will certainly continue this theme by developing a physical symptom in her body. Instead of pointing to the primary emotional source of this problem, a typical medical doctor would advise her to continue in some compensating sport. This will naturally bring improvement to her symptoms, at least as long as she practices her sport. However, her true problem will continue to wait patiently for resolution.

The problem becomes even more apparent for those athletes with mountains of muscle that seem to have grown beyond them. A primary example of this is bodybuilding. The bodybuilder's case is similar to the *athletic heart.* Its medical term is *hypertrophic muscles,* meaning "muscles that have grown excessively." The muscle-bound person apparently desires to look strong—and so he does. Nevertheless, the question remains as to whether he really is strong. As is generally known, true strength lies within, where it is not obvious. The suspicion is that something lavishly cultivated on the physical level is compensating for what is missing or neglected in the emotional life.

Most sports which are performed to excess are substitutes for a neglected emotional aspect. Of course, this does not always relate to the heart and only a small fraction of sports really lead to cardiac enlargement. Long-distance runners are the classic example, whereby their sport practically transforms them into lonesome high-performance machines. They run silently for mile after mile, usually racing only against themselves and the clock, as they say with pride. The Czech Emil Zatopek, also called "the Locomotive," had a legendary reputation for being such a runner. If one considers how a person can gain so much "pleasure" out of this sport, one may be able to comprehend the character of such extreme hobbies. A person with an overflowing heart—who heartily seeks the company of other people and would like to clasp them all to his heart, who laughs in a heartwarming manner and joyfully gives his heart away—probably looks for a hobby that is less hearty than marathon running. The historical example of the original runner at the Battle of Marathon who collapsed and died at his destination is characteristic of this extreme. One does not need to be an internist to diagnose heart failure in such a case.

The opposite extreme (the heart that is too small) is the product of a lack of challenge for the body. The owner of such a heart is also unaware that she is failing to challenge her own center and so the heart must express this problem physically in lieu of true awareness. However, the heart that is too small only emerges as a medical problem indirectly, such as in low blood pressure and in resulting circulatory problems. After all, blood pressure that is too low requires that the heart do less work than expected and so the organ suffers a lack of challenge. Not challenging the heart enough in the figurative sense means that it faces too small a requirement—too little courage, strength, love, and emotion. This lack of emotional challenge, which in reality means too little demand on the heart, in turn remains unconscious. It sinks from potential consciousness into the shadow and manifests itself as a physical symptom in the form of a heart that is too small—resulting in an inadequate blood pressure.

Smallness and weakness are the themes that people with small hearts must resolve, just as people with cardiac enlargement must resolve the theme of size, strength, and progress from a large heart to big-heartedness. In the process, unresolved faint-heartedness can develop into conscious caution and true modesty, while unresolved weakness can become genuine devotion.

Once again, a certain amount of conscious effort is necessary for a person not to be bound to the opposite extreme. The person with the heart that is too large must naturally also learn modesty and devotion at some point. The theme of size and weight—which the body has shown to be a priority—is the most important at the moment. If a person can express his big-heartedness in an emotional manner and can acknowledge the importance to his heart that his destiny seems to demand of him, it is the right time and much easier to resolve the opposite pole. Naturally, something similar applies to the other side. If the person with the small heart has accepted his primary themes of personal modesty and devotion and has begun to put them consciously into practice, the themes of strength and big-heartedness also demand resolution. After the realization of his personal tasks, he will have a much easier time conquering the opposite pole in any case.

The typical gender distribution of both of these problems, which we encounter again in the section dealing with abnormal blood pressure, illustrates another characteristic of our society on the level of the heart. While men in our society have difficulties finding their inner strength, their power, and their ability to consciously stand tall, women tend to have a problem with conscious devotion and accepting the surrender required for any type of true development in the religious-spiritual sense.

3. Constrictions of the Heart

3.1 Angina Pectoris—The Narrow Heart

The word *angina* already suggests the fear associated with this syndrome. It means *narrowness.* Consequently, angina pectoris is the narrowing of the chest and the morphological basis for this is the constriction of the heart or the blood vessels supplying it. The term *narrow-mindedness* (narrow-heartedness) speaks for itself.

Almost unbearable pain distinguishes an angina pectoris attack, which can transform itself to a sensation of impending doom, and so approaches the intensity of a heart attack. Such episodes often do evolve into heart attacks. The description for this pain is usually a life- threatening sensation of constriction and fear, as the heart seems to be contracting convulsively as if an iron fist were clenching it. The pain typically begins behind the sternum and radiates upward from it into the left shoulder and the left arm. If it lasts longer than a quarter of an hour, it may quite possibly be a heart attack. Within a few minutes, the entire left upper side of the body up to the nape of the neck and even to the larynx can be in pain. Since we understand that pain is an alarm signal, a type of cry for help, it is the left and, therefore,

Constrictions of the Heart

the feminine side of the upper body that is calling for help. Apparently, this area urgently needs attention.

One can divide the course of the angina pectoris attack into roughly two phases. In the beginning stage of the illness, the heart cries for help through its expression of pain, which stands in the foreground; the patient feels excited, afraid, and worried. He wants fresh air and actively seeks out help. This stage is often still a functional, spasmodic constriction of the coronary vessels. At this point, the heart is caught in a virtual headlock as the patient fights actively for release. This wrestling allusion from the days of childhood is also quite appropriate because the feminine, childlike softness and heartfelt areas are under pressure. In contrast, the serious attack in the progressive second stage forces the victim to stop all strenuous activities at once, whether they are physically or emotionally strenuous. The patient must rest. Rest seems to be what is most lacking at the moment and as a general trend of recent behavior. The physical reason for this is obvious. In terms of the heart tissue, angina pectoris signals inadequate circulation, which indicates nothing more than malnutrition on a basic level. The heart does not receive enough nourishment. This purely physical state already reveals a psychosomatic double meaning. In such a situation, the body takes its only chance to rest completely and lowers its energy consumption as much as possible. Such resting is an attempt to take it easy through life because in all other cases the body will promptly strike the narrow boundaries of its heart.

These boundaries are the walls of the coronary vessels which are constricted and have sometimes already hardened. Recent studies show that spasmodic constrictions of physically healthy heart muscles can lead to angina pectoris attacks. This is easy to understand with respect to the principle of the conservation of energy (described at the beginning of this book). If a person closes up during a conversation or conflict (because he must subconsciously block a certain topic that has touched his heart) this energy must enter the body. Then it will manifest itself in the coronary vessels, which close themselves and become cramped. At a minimum, the patient receives an impression of his own withdrawal. Frequently forcing the body into this substitute role is correspondingly forcing it to have functional vascular spasms and the danger increases for physical damage to the vessels. Raised blood pressure—the imperative consequence of constricted vessels—is one of the most important risk factors for arteriosclerosis. However, calcification of the coronary vessels (coronary sclerosis) is nothing more than arteriosclerosis in a particularly important region of the body.

The layman's expression, *arterial calcification,* only refers to the final stage of the disease, since a disease process has preceded it in the arterial walls for a number of years; calcium actually plays no role in this. The beginning of the disease causes damage to the *intima*—the sensitive layer of the artery. In recent times, an abrupt increase in blood pressure has been identified as the primary cause of the initial—still minimal—tearing in the inner wall lining of the blood vessels. In the next step, this completely asymptomatic damage offers various fatty substances (lipids and especially cholesterol) the opportunity to deposit themselves. Gradually, these deposits thicken until finally they jut out in spurs from the artery walls as *plaque.* In this stage the bloodstream can already be blocked—especially if its related basic emotional situation continues to exist. If the vessels now act as substitutes for emotional constriction, they have even less latitude and heart trouble is much more likely to result. Such deposits can "calcify" over time and thereby harden (sclerosis). Although sclerotic vessels no longer experience constant deviations and increases in blood pressure, they slowly lose their flexibility. If this process progresses further, the blood supply to the heart becomes increasingly poor. In this case, the danger for angina pectoris and heart attack is greatly increased as well.

In addition, these deposits form the basis for a number of dangerous complications. It might happen that the plaque surface becomes rough and so blood clots can become form. Blood clots not only contribute to obstructing a vessel but can be torn away and, in the form of embolisms, block the arteries which are further upstream. Such blood clot obstructions have the medical epithet *thrombosis* at the site of their formation, and they are called *embolism* at the place where they deposit.

In Western industrial nations, more than half of all men over the age of forty-five already have plaque in their coronary arteries. The high level of female hormone (estrogen) protects women to a large degree from coronary sclerosis during their fertile years. This also indicates that the neglected feminine part of the psyche tends to express itself in the hardening of the cardiac supply vessels. In the reverse, practiced femininity seems to prevent coronary sclerosis—as a hormone on the physical level or as emotions on the archetypal level. After menopause, women quickly catch up to men in damage to the coronary vessels. Society's modem domination by the masculine element shifts increasingly into the lives of women.

The handicaps that result from heart disease are less conspicuous in our culture, merely because of the widespread lack of exercise. The heart is enormously flexible and it may even be able to compensate for reduced vascular volume of more than fifty percent so that the heart can still have enough blood. On the other hand, this also shows the alarming extent of the problem that may have already occurred when pain occurs during strain. Regrettably, this is often the late point in time when many affected people first think about their hearts.

Even a straightforward description of these physical occurrences can create an emotional resonance because body and soul are so closely connected, a fact that language describes in its psychosomatic form. The second phenomenon after pain (already encountered in angina pectoris) is constriction. Feeling constriction is the first physical sensation. The victim is naturally unaware of the purpose of this figurative narrow-heartedness. An aware person would not have to sink into his psychological shadow and emerge with a physical symptom. After all, the task and the virtue of a symptom are to project the problem onto the screen of the body and so induce understanding in the patient. Therefore, the manifested symptom is proof that the patient misunderstood the meaning of the message and is far from accepting it.

The oppressive feeling that accompanies every attack clearly indicates the tight spot that has ensnared the patient unawares. The heart contracting convulsively in one's chest embodies the cramping and struggling of repressed matters of the heart.

A victim of hardening *(sclerosis* from the Greek *sklerds,* meaning *hard)* feels the hard beating of his distressed heart—as if a stone were in his chest. The final phase of this development is an actually petrified heart; the "calcification" (stone) that burdens the heart makes life difficult for the patient.

Medical research rounds off this picture by proving that this vehement pain—possibly as intense as a sensation of impending doom—results from an inadequate supply of essential elements to the heart. The heart is starving and it no longer receives sufficient energy to survive. The symbolic heart also receives no nourishment. Constriction and shortage strangle it, as if it were a besieged fortress with its elixir of life drained away. The sense of impending doom and the fear of death hardly require any further interpretation. The threat of physical destruction is imminent, and one's fear is well founded. However, that the patient himself is guilty of slowly strangling his own heart by not giving it enough nourishment and attention, is a concept quite foreign to him. If it were familiar to the patient, his heart would never have had to utter such desperate screams of pain in the first place.

Symptoms reveal the problems to a patient in rich symbolic images and they also precisely describe the location of the problem. A person threatened by frequent and serious angina pectoris attacks must constantly live in fear of the next heart attack, and therefore he must adjust his entire life to his heart condition. This is precisely the symbolic issue. All other needs must come second to the hard and painful demands of the heart—rest and relaxation. Even a person who never before listened to the voice of the heart must pay undivided attention. The heart frequently says some very painful things, since it has usually suffered neglect for years, which is especially true in moments when he

Constrictions of the Heart

had closed himself and his heart with particularly strong resolution. During these moments, the coronary vessels close up and thereby attract attention. The heart, once again, is the center of life—however, in a figurative sense, it is the physical heart that is replacing the emotional heart.

The pain of angina pectoris channels one's attention to heartaches and to the left, feminine, side of the upper body. The problem emanates from the heart, but in its course it also radiates out to the entire feminine side of one's being. By nature, men usually have greater difficulty coming to terms with their feminine side (anima) than women. No wonder women in the years between their first menses and menopause find extended protection against angina pectoris while most are strongly experiencing their femininity. Women apparently tend less to narrow heartedness or, stated more positively, they are more generous of heart.

Resulting suggestions for therapy seem quite obvious, but it is important to follow the correct steps carefully and in order. Naturally, constriction needs expansion and hardness should take on more softness. For example, a withdrawn person with a petrified heart would find it very relieving to cry from deep within the heart. Such a person immediately resists this suggestion by saying that he has not cried for a long lime, and he cannot even remember the last time it happened. He will counter further that he has no reason to cry and would not even know how to find such a reason. This attitude is appropriate in his situation since the preceding step is still missing.

Even if the patient were gently but firmly forced to take this second step, he could still not solve his problem, which is evident from experiments in orthodox medicine. According to allopathic thought, the constriction of coronary vessels can expand by means of violence. The most common medication for the treatment of an angina pectoris attack is explosive nitroglycerine. Taken as needed, these little red capsules blast open the constricted coronaries. However, they do not touch the fundamental problem. The solution does not become clear to the patient, nor can it prevent or reduce the chances of a future attack. Balloon catheters inserted into the veins can push open narrowed passages and the relief lasts longer than with nitroglycerine, but the underlying problem remains unattended. The patient will soon return to the same dead-end or his cleared vessel will re-clog, if he does not use the time he has bought for essential, inner steps. In a bypass operation, a piece of the patient's leg vein becomes a diversion (or bypass) for the narrowed pathways, which postpones the problem but does not solve it. If the victim does not take the entire matter to heart emotionally, the bypass will quickly re-close. A closed heart can only be opened briefly by mechanical measures, while chemical remedies (nitrates) only help for some ten minutes. The only lasting solution must occur on the emotional level. A person who takes nothing more to heart than the surgeon's knife will remain dependent on the surgeon. A heart that does not open voluntarily from within cannot remain open and wide for long—even with the most sophisticated surgeries.

A person must find the "key" before she can open her heart, and this key is the perception of her own situation. She must recognize and accept her situation for what it is—a dead-end—which gives her a chance to return to action. Someone whose constricted, cramped heart takes a breather through attacks of pain stands with her back against the wall. This is what she must first admit to herself Her life will stop if she does not become concerned with this problem. The honest diagnosis and advice of an internist can be an important contribution to this step of self-knowledge. The next step is to take inventory of the problem—to study the wall. The building blocks of this wall are evident in the symbolic language of the body. A person will discover unpleasant things about herself—nearly as frightening as that constricting fear of angina pectoris. If this were not so, she would not have had to repress anything. The fact that one had to repress anything at all reveals what alarm and danger one felt. Somebody who is not involved might view these issues as harmless, but this is unimportant here. The symptoms always carry the most difficult lesson for the victim himself. In each case, it is the greatest challenge that destiny has to offer him at that time.

Recognizing the meaning of a symptom is certainly much more difficult than the first step, which merely required an honest evaluation about one's life expectancy. A new openness in lifestyle and way of living is now a must. A person is often incapable of such revealing honesty when he confronts the phenomenon, which is regrettably well-known as being blind where the self is concerned. Nearly everyone is afflicted with this blindness when it comes to their own life, which is why self-knowledge is one of the greatest challenges to which a person can aspire.

Yet the next step requires even greater inner strength since it means recognizing and accepting unpleasant perceptions. This step is to acquiesce to the symptom that may have already been torture for a long time. The body's message is justified and fitting and deep acceptance is the only way to create a reliable foundation for future changes. This requires the recognition that the symptom is not an accident but is rather an appropriate occurrence in accordance with certain laws. Every symptom belongs to its owner; it is completely in the right place and in its own element. It exacted payment which was entirely due. If one views the entire drama as a whole, with all its entanglements, the symptom seems to be the best thing that could have happened to the patient, a fact that is naturally easier for an outsider to see than for the affected person himself. The process may be long (but necessary) before the patient can learn to share this opinion. There are no substitutes for this path. It cannot complete its destiny as long as the patient feuds with fate.

After the patient has mastered thankful acceptance of the symptom and its message, the necessary opportunities will follow as a result of the body communicating with the conscious mind. "Sorely tried by illness" is an expression that reveals much wisdom. A person can only pass this kind of test by accepting the situation, perceiving its purpose, and reacting to it appropriately. The patient will not see any sense in changing the problem at issue until she reaches this point. There is also the obvious danger in aiming impetuously for the opposite pole which for angina-pectoris patients would be "looking for space" after much constriction and suffering in the heart. This is not the right time for such a reaction and if the patient chooses to act too soon, it could definitely lead to her flight from the real issue.

An impatient desire to act in an opposite manner indicates the wish to escape from the old, unpleasant pole as quickly as possible. Physical and emotional hardness of heart is naturally very unpleasant and when the patient recognizes his plight, he understandably longs for softness. On the other hand, it is precisely the principle concealed in the hardness or any other manifestation of the symptom with which such a person has difficulty. Every symptom *embodies* such a principle—even though it is naturally far from being resolved. Dealing with the very principles or archetypes facilitates the discovery of this principle behind the symptom.

To the angina-pectoris patient, this requires finding the red thread that runs through the symptoms, constriction, hardness, withdrawal, and oppression. People who are familiar with the original principles will immediately recognize the influence of the Saturnian archetype as represented in mythology by Cronos-Saturn. It manifests itself as angina pectoris in its least resolved and therefore most painful form. Other symptoms—the restriction of circulatory pathways, loss of vitality, insufficient nourishment to the heart, fear of death—belong to this principle and so are a part of the lessons the patient must take on. One must first learn to reconcile one principle before progressing to the lesson to be learned from the opposite principle.

The answer to the question: "What does this symptom cause me to do?" frequently offers help in identifying the next lesson. It puts the angina-pectoris patient in his place. Such initial activity reflects the heart's desperate search for outside help while in its advanced stage it requires that he forsake all external activities and interests to concentrate on the heart. Just as the heart concentrates on the most essential thing in this situation (namely survival) the patient must learn to concentrate on his center and

Constrictions of the Heart

the truly essential things in life. Concentration and limitation are the lessons to be learned, which are both more sensible modes of behavior for the affected principle than the previous approach of constriction and deficiency. Just as the heart must now manage with the bare necessities, so must the patient do likewise. He will find what is truly necessary in his center—the place where the core of his character is concentrated. This also means that he must find the essence of his problem. If he faces the hard core of his own truth with determination, he will do justice to the principle of hardness on a resolved level. Besides inner peace, as a replacement for forced heart convalescence, the patient may achieve a certain stillness in the outer processes instead of in the coronary vessels, and this process offers the opportunity to embrace contemplation and find the way back to one's own heart.

The affected person will discover a series of emotions that match the constriction and hardness of the symptoms very well and that he has not previously admitted to himself We must consider fear and hatred in the primary positions here as well as those emotions that are associated with narrowness and withdrawing. Fear and narrowness originate from the same linguistic source (from the Latin *angustus* meaning narrow). In addition, physical constriction accompanies all situations of fear. The chest becomes tight and the breathing and the vessels become more constricted, which explains why a person also has "cold feet" and hands in a situation connected to fear, or feels "a chill down his spine."

Hate correlates with withdrawal and the opposite pole can best illustrate this. Hate is in contrast to love, but we already equated love with openness and expansiveness. It is open to everything and wants to let everything in. Conversely hate leads to limitation, exclusion, and struggle.

Fear and hate first need to find recognition and expression instead of being pressed down into the heart. As soon as the angina-pectoris patient achieves this, he can concern himself with becoming free of hatred; he can learn to love. Before the patient can open up to other people and to other feelings, he will have to open up to his own emotions. This means nothing less than learning how to recognize and love those feelings.

Attacks of pain also point in a similar direction. Instead of hurting one's own heart, the patient must learn to take the field (where required) against those who actually should be confronted. Inevitably, the entire symptom forces him to direct his attention to his heart and he must consider the entire left (feminine) side of his body as well. This can also occur by his own resolve to do so, instead of pain forcing him to act. Anyone who listens to the refined expressions of the feminine part of the soul and has an open ear for the more tender impulses of the heart does not need heart-rending screams of pain to roar at him. However, the *open ear* that listens attentively to the inner life—to one's own center—belongs to the affected original principle, as does the necessary obedience.

This last point automatically leads the patient to reconcile with the opposite pole—becoming opened and expansive to other people and to other needs. On the basis of the previous steps, this happens quite naturally; the new attitude fails into the open lap as if it were a piece of ripe fruit. A person who has created order within and around herself, who is on good terms with herself and her hardness (which she has transformed into steadiness and resoluteness) can also more easily open up and love. She no longer needs to fear any physical symptoms because they merely reflect inner problems. There is certainly a reason for the first Christian commandment: "Love your neighbor as yourself." If (according to the definition of love) one replaces the word *love* with the words *open to,* a comprehensive harmony with the Christian message results. This would also create harmony with the second Christian commandment that is just as important: "Love your enemies." The enemies of the (angina-pectoris) patient are the symptoms. Learning to love them and their deciphered message means to open oneself up; in this manner the symptoms become friends on the path of personal evolution.

3.2 Heart Attack—The Breaking Heart

The heart attack has many names and, above all, it has achieved a regrettable popularity in recent decades. From heart attack and heart failure to the medical expressions of *myocardial* or *cardiac infarction,* acute coronary occlusion or myocardial necrosis, all of these terms describe the same phenomenon. Despite the different names, the syndrome is usually quite distinct and striking. The symptoms of an angina pectoris attack can become very intense and so the patient can hardly remain calm; the pain is too fierce and life-threatening. The infarction pains begin under the sternum and radiate out into the left upper body and arm as with angina pectoris, but they may even reach into the upper abdominal region. More than half of the heart attacks start in the same way as an angina pectoris attack but the symptoms do not subside and they become increasingly intense. They last for more than a quarter of an hour—possibly even for hours or days. Since the explosive nitroglycerine capsules provide no relief in this case, one can practically consider the medication to be a diagnostic criterion. One can understand this by examining the basis of the problem. These pains are no longer the warning cries of a starving heart but are the death screams and struggles of the already strangled part of the heart. The destroyed muscle tissue corresponds to the typical sensation of impending doom that accompanies the fear of death. One out of five heart-attack patients dies during this acute stage. The prognosis is largely dependent on the localization and the extent of the necrotic (dead) tissue and the reserves that the heart possesses. If the tissue destruction is too extensive, the affected person must share in the destruction along with it. As the center and capital of the physical body, the heart becomes a necropolis, a city of the dead.

In addition to the symptoms already familiar from angina pectoris, there are a series of apparently senseless physical reactions.

For example, the patient becomes restless and very active at a time when he needs nothing more than peace and quiet. However, the body has exceeded its possibilities to compensate in this near-death situation and simply has no control any longer. Overstrained, it reacts accordingly with nausea, vomiting, profuse sweating, and other such symptoms.

One may also experience similar difficulties in comparatively harmless situations in which overstraining occurs. One example is seasickness. In this case, the eyes report a calm situation to the central headquarters because they truly cannot perceive any movement of the ship from beneath the deck. Yet, at the same time, the vestibular system of the inner ear transmits intense rolling motions to the same central headquarters which, in turn, no longer knows whom to trust. In its dilemma, the body will typically become nauseated because it does not want to accept what its sensory organs perceive. As a result, the liquid in the middle ear spins around, and the person vomits.

With seasickness, the organism gradually learns that in this case it cannot trust its eyes. With a heart attack, the body is subjected to much more extensive strain by what it must now perceive. All of its reactions are directed towards survival and are based on the availability of adequate reserves. It may further increase the blood pressure within the failing system and thereby make the situation in the body even worse in the long run. With this response, the body indicates that it is under the utmost pressure, but there is no authority to answer to this information. This also applies in the situation when the body attempts to restimulate the heart and actually stimulates the dying organ to a galloping rhythm. A large portion of all heart attacks are associated with such rhythm problems, which is a further indication that the central point has lost balance and nothing remains to keep even a trace of order.

Returning to the metaphor of the heart as the body's capitol, we can ascertain that everything is in complete chaos in the city's structure. The coordination has gone and specific areas have suffered destruction while other areas are trying to solve the overall problem. They try to help compensate by doing the work of the failing cells, but they often just do not have the ability to do so. In this condition, much depends on whether or not the city had made provisions for such emergencies during better times (for example, by practicing crisis drills—thereby also training various departments to substitute for each other). Sport can be such a preparation for the heart. Physical effort makes demands on the heart and trains it for difficult supply situations by developing parallel circulatory systems. This means that more than one vessel can supply blood to particularly strained areas of the heart and so the vessels are not as indispensable.

If one equates an angina pectoris attack to an extended labor strike, or even a general strike in the case of a major attack, an emergency situation with irreparable damage occurs when it comes to a heart attack. The circumstances become especially precarious if important connections in the central information- conduction system try to run through the now blocked and destroyed area. This is frequently the case for a heart attack in the region of the right coronary artery, the vessel that supplies oxygenated blood to the posterior wall of the heart and consequently also to the sinoatrial and AV nodes. It is possible that a small part of a backyard can collapse in the city and even a such small collapse might strike the central, vital nerve to the entire city and consequently paralyze an entire country. In such situations, the nerves can easily start to flutter and the cardiac nerves are not immune to this either. If the heart begins to flutter, the situation is very threatening and yet an emergency procedure continues to function. Although the rhythm has given way to chaos, life grasps at the last straw—even in this hopeless situation. It manages to limp along as best it can from the small amount of blood still supplied to the heart in the midst of the collapse. However, if the central cardiac nerves begin to break down completely and defibrillate, there will be no further supply of blood. In a state of absolute superexcitation, the heart remains oddly calm as the blood pressure drops to zero and the circulatory system stops along with it. Death occurs due to heart failure.

Heart-Aches

When life has reached its last moments, it offers a grotesque illustration of the exaggerated and the excessive manifestation of life. Everything is still laboring at top speed but there is no supervision to coordinate it and so it labors uselessly. The unifying main idea that integrated all of the meaningful activities from the central point—that directed them to the common goal—has gone. This also describes the psychological situation of the typical candidate for a heart attack shortly before the collapse. Death is already standing at the threshold, waiting only for an opportunity to enter as the patient still toils and slaves on behalf of things that are irrelevant in the truest sense of the word—things that have become completely disconnected from the central problem. When death enters, it has usually already been knocking for quite some time, as a zealous attitude had deliberately ignored the knocking. When death strikes it is a surprise for the afflicted person—perhaps also for the patient's relatives who had mistaken the body's exaggerated frenzied state for life, even though death had been lurking for a long while. The desperate last struggle forces the inwardly driven person even more certainly into death's arms.

In addition to the heart's fluttering and fibrillation, Father Death finds other entrances during the heart attack. The most drastic entry in every respect is the actual physical breaking of the heart, a condition the medical profession calls *myocardial rupture*. This occurs when the area of the heart attack is so massive that the surrounding heart tissue cannot supplant the enormous pressure for the dead area during the systole. The lifeless area of the cardiac wall gives way—or the blood that is under high pressure burrows into it. A rupture in the heart occurs and blood pours out into the heart sac. There is no chance for such a torn heart (and its owner) to survive. On the one hand, the torn heart can no longer pump blood, as the *nectar of life* seeps out from it in the truest sense of the word. On the other hand, the blood that has penetrated the heart sac suffocates the heart from the outside. The pericardium (the skin of the heart sac) is so inelastic that the exuded blood can no longer escape. As a

Constrictions of the Heart

result, the pressure from outside the heart increases with every additional heartbeat. The heart either strikes itself dead or becomes a victim of its own corruption. In this case, death enters so quickly that the medical profession calls it a sudden death. In contrast, a common phrase that people will say is "A heart attack that has claimed yet another victim."

If the cardiac wall does not break but only gives way a bit more to the blood pressure, a ballooning of the cardiac wall occurs. Medical science calls this an *aneurysm*. The heart remains permanently expanded at this spot, but the stretched and expanded part no longer participates in the contraction work, since it has died. The heart and its owner remain considerably handicapped; even though the patient may survive the heart attack, the afflicted spot later forms a scar. The expansion of the heart is a task in the symbolic sense. If a person refuses expansion on the emotional level, then it will shift to the physical level and a symptom will definitely result—in this case it is particularly unpleasant and dangerous.

A further complication of the heart attack that sometimes occurs is an embolism. The chaos resulting from the tissue collapse also affects the flow of blood. The blood normally passes through the heart in a very orderly fashion and, despite the high speed and high pressure, heavy turbulence and swirling now take place. However, in this situation the blood tends to coagulate and thereby cause thrombosis. Such blood clots can travel to all areas of the body where they obstruct the vessels and cause major problems for their victim. The resulting supply and congestion problems naturally worsen a circulatory situation that is already tense enough. The congestion burdens the heart even further and so even if the heart can maintain its emergency service, it cannot manage the entire volume of blood that usually flows through during better times. Since the heart attack usually affects only the left heart or its left ventricle, the congestion affects the lung. The blood that the heart has not adequately transported begins to build up in the lungs and, finally, if the lung vessels have no more capacity to hold this blood, it exudes from the pulmonary alveoli (air cells). Difficulties in breathing are the usual result and they can develop to extreme shortness of breath. The lungs become saturated by blood-fluid, a condition the medical profession calls pulmonary *edema*.

The physical basis of a heart attack principally corresponds to that of the angina-pectoris attack. However, the obstructed flow in the affected coronary arteries is more serious. The circulatory emergency lasts until the dependent myocardial tissue has died. The heart attack usually comes from a long build up of coronary sclerosis, a condition for which the victim has received ample warning, and so finally his narrow-heartedness has been forced to confront him in a physical manner. However, a heart attack can develop (this occurs less frequently) without much previous damage preparing the way and would usually happen as the result of an emotionally constricted situation.

Whatever causes the acute circulatory emergency is unimportant to the final consequences; a thrombosis of the coronary artery is the usual reason for a heart attack. We will delve even more extensively into thrombosis symbolism in the section concerning "The Organic Language of the Circulatory System." For now, it is adequate to say that the blood, as a symbol of life energy, loses its fluid properties and becomes solidified. Something that was flowing has turned into a lump, which threatens the heart. With the solidification of a liquid—the coagulation of something that was flowing—one is on the track of a well- known phenomenon. "Everything flows," said Heraclitus, who was referring to life on this earth. When something gets stuck and no longer moves, it distances itself from life and approaches death. The theme of hardening something that should be soft and flexible has already appeared in the earlier description of sclerosis of coronary vessels; the same principle restates itself for the heart attack. The hardening of the vascular wall and the increasing brittleness create the condition which allows blood clots to form.

In contrast to angina pectoris, in the event of a heart attack the aspect of dying has to be considered. Even if the patient survives, part of the heart has died. Something dead is at his very center from now on, and he bears a scar as a reminder of it. This is no longer a wound in the heart; this is something with a different quality—something that is dead. A certain amount of healing may admittedly take place, but it can only occur by relatively coarse scar tissue replacing vital muscle tissue. This scar tissue cannot fulfill the demands exerted on it in any way. The hardness and rigidity of the scar tissue is a symbolic reminder that in emergency repair work something vital and highly alive can only be replaced by relatively lifeless material.

The fear of death also accompanies the physical event of a heart attack on the emotional level; this terror makes the relevant theme more than clear. Even if the afflicted person does survive, he still has allowed something to die irrevocably within himself. The patient has parted with an area of the heart; nothing but an inferior substitution can be left behind in its place. This experience ranks among the worst feelings—probably the worst—that a person can have; this is not merely obvious—one should take this to heart. The victim usually is forced to experience the death of his heart—piece by piece—with full consciousness and an otherwise living body. At best, the patient will be incomplete for his remaining life.

An outsider cannot comprehend the emotional collapse that accompanies the breaking of the heart. However, it frequently leads to the impressive development of the stricken patient. Afterwards, it is usual for a heart-attack survivor to make more out of her remaining life than she previously did, when she still had a physically unlimited abundance of opportunities from which to choose. This primarily occurs if one is able to recognize, accept, and resolve the emotional limitations with which one has practically strangled one's live. The patient truly takes leave from a part of herself and through this step rediscovers her own identity. Many patients report this parting pain; nearly all of them have experienced their life after heart attack as a gift that they can feel joyful about in a way that had been unfamiliar to them before— an approach to life that they want to treat more consciously in the future. In this way, the heart attack frequently succeeds in something that even committed partners and therapists could not achieve—namely introducing a hard-core chain smoker to the pleasure of fresh air, motivating a couch potato to take pleasant walks, even convincing an overweight person to enjoy getting into shape. Although these external changes become the most obvious to one's environment, the inner transformations are even more substantial. The hardest business people suddenly discover that they have a heart for their family whose members had only existed on the sidelines before the heart attack. A person's center and the core of his own life often take on the central meaning that they always had on the physical level.

If the promise that the patients make to themselves is as fragile as their coronaries, they must expect some additional coaching from fate. It is highly probable that this might manifest itself as a new heart attack; if this is the case, it will certainly be an even harder lesson. Anyone who is not willing to meet his own inner center with a clear single-mindedness (which again is nothing other than resolved hardness) will have to suffer from the hardness in his own heart. Fate itself is not really hard, but it is more resolute than people are and therefore it will try to point to the problem even more clearly to the case of a repeat offender.

Because of its mechanistic picture of the world, orthodox medicine naturally has tried to investigate the conditions in the physical body that lead to the heart attack. As could be expected, medical science has been successful in putting the blame on cigarettes, lipids in the blood, excess salt, and a lack of exercise. However, even orthodox medicine has never been able to overlook the fact that emotional conditions decisively share involvement in the foundation of a heart attack. The very generalized term *stress* has become a synonym for largely unsettled emotional sources. Since the problem has grown during recent decades, an increasing number of medical professionals have come to see the emotional dimension as being more than just a fringe condition for a heart attack. The medical doctor and life analyst Condrau presents this viewpoint:

However, loneliness, as we know from experience, 'breaks the heart'.... The oppressive isolation of humanity finds its physical embodiment in cardiac pain. The heart, completely ignored up to that time, now begins to speak. This also shows that metaphors have a very essential significance that goes far beyond the symbolic. The language of the heart is a true language, and the metaphor is more than merely a parable.[7]

Inspired by the earlier work of Alexander, research on the emotional basis for constrictions of the coronary vessels has increased. Researchers eventually discovered a personality profile typical of heart-attack patients. It is not at all surprising that this list largely correlates with the picture of the high blood pressure patient since this is one of the most important risk factors for coronary constriction. Before taking a closer look at this type-A personality pattern, it is important to point out that such typecasting must always be viewed as a generalization. The more sharply such generalizations define a situation, the more abstract they become with respect to a specific case. As a result of this process, they often become inaccurate when applied to the individual. In contrast, the more diverse the analysis, considering each of the various sub-types, the more blurred and less general is its message. Therefore, interpreting the specific symptoms of a particular person can result in an accurate picture and one with greater certainty.

The type-A human being (named with the first letter of the alphabet by the Americans Rosenmann and Friedmann in 1966) bears the characteristic of always striving to be the first. This person feels driven to gel ahead by a strong pressure for success and performance. It also drives him to compete with his fellow human beings for the sake of corporate and social recognition. He puts himself and other people under pressure as he strives for complete control over himself and his environment.

He subjects himself and his life to one goal—dominance. Involved in many ways, he feels concerned with a number of things at one time; this schedule makes him pressed for time and contributes to his impatient nature. Relaxation becomes almost impossible. Although he can be completely successful in realizing his high and broad goals with the help of his unusual potential for aggression, he tends to feel dissatisfied with himself and his world. Parallel to his aggressive ways, he permits himself a distinct aversion to conflict in terms of topics that are important and, above all, related to himself. The reason for this lies in his great fear of criticism and failure; the troublesome consequence is dangerously pent-up aggression. He compensates for his missing self-esteem with a constant willingness to perform and the philosophy that a person has to earn everything by himself alone, without any exceptions. According to the German motto "what you have is what you are," he strives for status symbols; he feels that it is important to be able to afford everything society has to offer. Precisely because of his forced, practically compulsive efforts to look good and make everyone happy, other people experience him as constricted and characteristically rigid.

On the other hand, he possesses an impressive intellectual and physical flexibility; however, this is in sharp contrast to his inhibitions about formulating his own emotional needs and expressing his feelings. This is a type of person who strives in an upward direction to the highest degree, but attaches only little importance to his emotional problems. All of this does not exactly predestine him to be a sick outsider in our performance-oriented society. Quite to the contrary, he is a popular achiever. In other words, the society prefers and practically encourages such heart-attack candidates. This is in no way surprising; the unconditional performance-oriented society naturally requires willingness to perform. We live, so to speak, in a type-A society in which everyone wants to be first. Since everyone cannot be in first place, it is obvious that difficulties and problems will arise. The dissatisfaction that this generates (which is called frustration these days) is naturally a further characteristic of the type-A personality. He therefore tends to display an irritated, annoyed mood and a constant attitude, which expects success to still come his way so that he will be number one. Since he constantly wants something and desires more of everything, an oddly unnatural and tense politeness becomes conspicuous in his behavior.

Life is an uninterrupted competitive event for him; he constantly engages this competition anew with a sense of ambition and responsibility. Nevertheless, his victories cannot provide any relief—no victory will ever exist that is going to make him happy. Each victory provides a short-lived thrill and it becomes the incentive for achieving even more within the shortest time possible, while the actual objective remains oddly unclear. It remains forever tantalizing in the far distance. His competitive approach to other contenders in the struggle for existence and his aggressive ambition that only knows how to "get ahead," but experiences not a single quiet moment of contemplation, drives the type- A into social isolation. His inability to open emotionally intensifies this and he compensates with cynicism. The result is a loneliness that he might or might not admit.

According to Lynch[8] this loneliness is one of the "most important causes of premature death." He writes, "Medical statistics on the loss of human relationships, lack of love, and human loneliness quickly reveal that the expression *broken heart* is not only a poetic image for loneliness and despair; it is also an overwhelming medical reality. All the necessary data indicates that the lack of human company, constant loneliness, social isolation, and the sudden loss of a beloved person are among the main causes for premature death."

On the one hand, there is also a great amount of documented material available on the emotional characteristics of heart-attack patients; on the other hand, there is an abundance of individual symptoms associated with the heart attack known to promote or complicate it. The interpretation of the latter can become the connecting link between the two levels. Excessively excited activity has already made an impression in the physical occurrence of the heart attack; one can also detect it in the preceding phase. The heart works at top speed while in the most blatant case—during the heart attack—it produces absolutely nothing. However, even in the previous time period, it had not succeeded in taking enough decisive action in comparison to the efforts it made. The hectic heart corresponds in this respect to its hectic owner who, despite all the (competitive) struggle, cannot achieve a decisive victory. Here the senseless actions of the heart attack are a striking reflection of the patient's feeling of pointlessness—often expressed verbally by heart attack candidates in therapeutic discussions. The heart no longer has any goal. Because of the absolute arrhythmia and, specifically, because of the fibrillation, the central concern has become lost in a chaos of individual actions. In a complete analogy, the owner has long been without a higher goal—the goal associated with the heart. In a flood of more or less individual actions, the central meaning in life has perished.

The theme of loneliness may be associated directly with the term cardiac infarction. *Infarcire* means *pressing into, or jamming,* and so the cardiac infarction is a "jamming" of the heart. When something has Jammed, nothing can go out and nothing can go in, which is exactly the problem in this case. No vital energy—no blood—enters those parts of the heart and the heart has permanently closed itself off. For quite some time the affected person has stopped allowing any feelings from the outside to enter the heart. Nothing has gone to his heart, nothing has touched his heart, and he has not even noticed it. The opposite is also true, as he has not released anything from his heart for a long time. He no longer speaks from his heart nor has he given heartfelt feelings free reign and allowed himself to be guided by his heart. Nothing in his life comes from the heart anymore. Quite the opposite has been true for some time, as the patient no longer speaks openly about his feelings. Yet, when a person can no longer speak from the heart and can no longer

Constrictions of the Heart

share anything (because he has withdrawn into his shell), his only choice is to be lonely.

The (unconscious) characteristic rigidity finds its symbolic expression in the hardening and inflexibility of the coronary vessels. Calcium plates armor the paths of vital energy and weigh them down, naturally obstructing the river of life—similar to the way in which a heavy knight's battle gear with its many armor plates may protect the knight from outside attacks but also impedes his movement and makes him inflexible. The armor makes its wearer impervious on one level and, as a result, he is very vulnerable on another level. Inside the hard, successful (competitive) fighter there is also a very vulnerable and sensitive child, just as a very timid being is inside the hard heart, barricaded with its calcium plates. Just as the knight seeks refuge in the constriction of his armor or fortress, there is also a constricted fear of being injured behind the heart barricades. On the emotional level, the usual cynicism creates an appropriate wall around one's own fearful existence. This emphasis on the borders through the patient's barricades and fortresses once again accentuates the demarcation and blockading of oneself which already characterizes the angina pectoris problem. Anyone who closes himself off has to exist in constricted circumstances and is naturally lonely.

The enormous physical performance expected of the heart reflects the equally enormous work output of the heart-attack candidate. Both are unable to permit themselves a breather and they are both under high pressure in the same way. The heart works against the high resistance of the constricted vessels while the heart-attack candidate works against the high resistance of the hostile environment, which is full of competitors and rivals who all want to be the winner. The person who tears himself apart for his work instead of developing his inner life should not be surprised if his heart breaks as well. To let himself be torn to pieces for the job, company, duties, and other responsibilities is a matter of choice and is an odd ideal nowadays. It receives an even more peculiar flavor when one remembers that one's own heart sometimes "falls to pieces" as well. Addiction to work is the most dangerous addiction of our time. In any case, it is much more common and more often fatal than other addictions usually singled out. Workaholics and alcoholics are definitely in the same boat in this society—even if they are at different ends of it.

The suppressed aggression of many people in danger of a heart attack is mirrored in the high stress in their vessels and the high pressure with which their blood is forced along its course. As with every other liquid under pressure, the pressed red *nectar of life* also has much energy bound within it. Just as the patients have difficulties directing their congested energy along the right paths and tend to let off steam in uncontrolled outbursts of fury and rage, the body can hardly translate this congested pressure energy into any productive sense. Instead, the body tends to express it in analogy and to create a way out by bursting vessels or even breaking the heart. These explosive and excessive pressure reactions contrast with the otherwise very controlled appearance of the patient. Just as they normally have everything well under control in life on the emotional and social level, their blood in the constricted and virtually concrete-encased or calcium-armored pipes that have replaced the living vessels are under particularly strict control. Small and large explosions have a ventilation function on both levels, as they show that one should not trust the flawless outer facade one bit.

One should not overlook the inability to relax deeply and to rest thoroughly—for this inability is a characteristic of heart-attack candidates. A heart that must constantly—day in, day out, year in, year out—work against the pressure that is doubly as high as planned, can no longer find any relaxation. It is also apparent that the vessels subject to high tension are not able to relax either. Just as high pressure is the basis of the cardiac infarction, so is the lack of relaxation.

3.3 Therapy for the Heart Attack

Therapy for the acute heart attack naturally belongs in the hands of orthodox medicine. However, it is customary in our culture that this attempt at healing takes place in an Intensive Care Unit, a choice which is still somewhat controversial. American studies have shown that the prospects are clearly better outside of intensive-care, provided that adequate treatment is available. With the use of the ECG and monitoring of the blood enzyme LDH (lactate dehydrogenase) one can quickly and reliably make a diagnosis. In addition, these measurements provide information on the localization and extent of the heart attack.

In terms of therapy, orthodox medicine first immobilizes the patient using chemical means. Because of the debilitating pain experienced in situations such as heart attacks, doctors usually prescribe morphine. As an external measure, they also prescribe confinement to bed, which is where the problem of intensive-care arises. The patient (with a life-threatening heart injury) will both actually and symbolically find the world of machines to be the worst conceivable condition for healing his painful heart.

Modem medicine can improve the state of the threatening circulatory collapse—both medicinally and through the infusion of additional fluids. Even if a severe circulatory shock has already occurred, it is possible to "bring back" the patient from the threshold of death. The administered medication revitalizes the arteries that have already given up. Furthermore, there are possible chemical approaches for relieving the existing vasospasms. Medicinal liquefaction of the blood prevents the danger of renewed clot formation. Even existing blood clots can sometimes be dissolved as a result. Medication can often favorably influence the larger problem of arrhythmia. Orthodox medicine still has a chance—even in the usually hopeless cases of heart fibrillation. The overly stimulated heart calms down by means of a strong electroshock with an external electrical force. Through this means it has the opportunity to at least find its way back to some sort of order.

The concrete and symbolic significance of these interventions is particularly suited to understanding the efficiency of the measures of orthodox medicine in these acute situations. Heart fibrillation is a situation in which the entire order in the electrical pulse generating system of the heart has broken down. Every cell transmits wild impulses but none of them can prevail and bring the others under its command to rouse them into mutual action. The hierarchy has collapsed. The heart is without leadership or has too many leaders who cannot agree. Because of their conflict, they are willing to let the whole thing come to an end. In this situation, the doctor intervenes and *with a single* (electrical) *stroke* deprives all the adversaries of their power. In the pause for rest that this creates, the pulse center that still is the strongest, even after everything it has been through recently, is given the opportunity to gather all the others behind it and take over leadership with its first stroke. This is how the intensive-care treatment helps the disoriented heart acquire a new hierarchy.

One can interpret other interventions in the same way. When a patient has already given up on himself so that, as a sign of this, the vessels of the circulatory system lose any kind of force of their own, the blood gets bogged down in the vessels and the circulation is brought to a standstill, he is injected with the stress hormone adrenaline which gets the circulation back on its feet once again. The doctor puts herself in the place of the adrenal gland as she stimulates the organism that is already giving in to resignation. A person's own adrenal gland is no longer capable of this, because it no longer has any reserves. The typical heart-attack patient lives in a constantly excited state with stress hormones above the normal level.

In the situation of a circulatory collapse, the inner strength of the patient is apparently no longer adequate to keep the body in line. The vital energy, symbolized by the blood, bogs down and comes to a standstill in the vessels. In this situation, the body receives fluid into the veins of the circulatory system directly from an infusion bottle. This fluid is an imitation of the cell water that the medical profession calls plasma expander because it stretches and expands the blood reserves. It fills the emptiness in a way that is also symbolically appropriate, for water is the classical symbol for the emotions. Therefore, the deficit in soul-energy is satisfied by an external source—at least symbolically. It is clear that the problem is specifically a lack of this water and, in this situation, no doctor would ever consider the idea of giving a blood transfusion. However, in terms of pure function, one could assume that blood would be an even better solution.

Once the circulation has come to a standstill, and blood clots have already closed a vessel in one section of the heart, there is a danger that fluids will solidify in other places and the flow will stop completely. The affected person no longer has the strength to keep the vital energy flowing. The doctor rescues him from this situation of overstrain by preventing any further coagulation chemically. This prevents the flow of life from being obstructed in other places by the clotting blood but it does not resolve the problems in the life circumstances of the patient. He is certainly obstinate in matters of the heart and, though his life has been saved temporarily, only some time has been won.

The administration of morphine also follows the same principle. At least on the material level, the doctor can temporarily satiate what is missing on the emotional level. In this current precarious situation such satisfaction can only be acquired in physical terms. The lack of inner peace that the patient suffers is life-threatening and is alleviated abruptly by the morphine. While this does not solve the problem, it does put it aside just for this moment of acute emergency. Biochemical inner peace is much better than none at all. The nervous distraction and the restless activity of the patient are typical of himself and of his life-style. This has brought him to the threshold of death, but it cannot become resolved in this extreme moment. The only remaining possibility is to flee to the opposite pole.

The situation is similar when a spasm of the coronary vessels leads to the final struggle for the heart. Once again, the allopathic concept governs this acute situation and the antispasmodic antidote leads to a state of relaxation. However, this relaxation cannot generally resolve the patient's problems in life. However, it can be instrumental in his present struggle for survival.

Therefore, orthodox medicine provides acute therapy for heart attacks in a very concerted effort. After the patient has survived the heart attack, these methods are just as inadequate as they are essential in the acute situation. The patient who can no longer get his river of life to flow on its own can find medicated relief from this chore until the end of his days. However, he will remain a cripple as a result and will resemble a person who always swims with a life jacket just because it saved his life at one point. He will simply lag behind in terms of his possibilities as a human being. If a person has to depend on antispasmodic remedies for relaxation and achieves calmness and inner peace through morphine and tranquilizers for all of his life, the problem becomes even more clear. Affected people seem to be running away from something. This 'something' is themselves or their learning task in life. In the previous examples, the respective medications are considered addictive drugs and therefore, these examples will quickly find agreement. Yet, the principle is no different for other medications such as the anticoagulants.

After the acute therapy that fate and orthodox medicine perform, the course must be set for the newly bestowed life. Medical science gets stuck at the level of phenomena. It is well documented that smoking damages the heart and vessels, and it is therefore shunned by medical experts. We do not consider the problem of why the patient smokes and, in due course, his situation drastically worsens. Obesity is treated in a similar manner. It has been determined to be a risk factor and is now taken care of by dieting. However, one hardly ever asks why the patient needs an entire body armor of fat in addition to the calcium artery armor. We use the same superficial, non psychological approach for dealing with blood pressure, salt consumption, high cholesterol, and lack of exercise. Whatever is too high is brought down using functional measures and whatever is too low is raised by the same types of methods. While the normal values celebrate their triumph, the affected patient remains a book sealed to himself and to the medical profession, and the heart attack is viewed as a terrible but senseless mishap because it is misunderstood.

Even with the most superficial reflection, it is obvious that these are not a collection of individual factors but an overall picture. It is a cycle of interdependent patterns, forming the inner pattern that made the heart attack necessary. This necessity can only be changed if the entire cycle is understood, preventing it from becoming a vicious circle. The type-A person lives in a very unstable equilibrium; it is not wise to take safety valves such as smoking and overeating away from him without a substitution. Patients frequently cannot renounce those habits without seriously endangering themselves, but fortunately in those cases they cannot do without them anyhow. The vicious circle that imprisons them also endangers them.

Every symptom, and naturally every addiction, has its purpose. It is only possible to give up the symptom when we can understand this purpose by means of some other technique. Otherwise, one creates a new, perhaps even more dangerous, symptom that conveys the same message. For example, if we forbid a smoking patient his vice, he could very well begin to eat more than his hunger demands and thereby create a new safety valve. However, this would be a new threat for his endangered heart and would hardly be an improvement. If a patient who smokes eats and drinks more than is necessary, he should not have all three vices taken away from him or, more accurately, have all three outlets plugged up, because it is quite possible that then a dangerous explosion of his aggressive energies will occur. Perhaps he will put up with the sacrifice for a time, but the longer he manages without, the greater the pressure becomes. We can now compare the patient to a steam kettle that has just had its high- pressure valve clogged up. It would be fatal to force the inner pressure to increase, particularly in the case of the heart-attack patient. The resulting kettle explosion can correspond to the next heart attack. What could more closely resemble the image of the kettle exploding as a result of high pressure than a heart bursting for the same reason?

Deep-reaching suggestions in therapy result in the same problem already seen for angina pectoris, namely the temptation to rescue oneself to the opposite pole because of a great aversion to the status quo. This is where deliverance is available, but only after one's own homework has been done. Before one can successfully learn a foreign language, one must first have a command of one's native language, even if this is a less spectacular challenge.

In essence, what has been said for angina pectoris also applies here because angina pectoris is a pre-cursor to a heart attack. However, now everything has been staged in a considerably more drastic and uncompromising light. If it was possible to help oneself before by reaching for the explosive capsules, now the person is helpless to the greatest degree and should be happy if it is not too late for any help at all. The demonstration of helplessness continues to take its course from the emergency physician taking over command at admission to the intensive-care unit. The go-getter has been very busy up until this moment as he was chasing after his ambitious goals without pause. All of his striving has been for domination and power and now he is helpless, in a symbolic sense, and sometimes unconscious, in a medical sense. The fallen hero of the performance-oriented society is similar to a knight in armor. He appears to be invincible and superior to everyone else in his shining armor, then suddenly he becomes helpless when he falls down and can no longer even stand up on his own. He must admit to his weakness and vulnerability; his circumstances very distinctly remind him of it.

Forced to his knees and, therefore, into a posture of humility, everything that had given him support has gone. This is humility in the face of death and he really has nothing left but his bare life. Reduced to this extremely desperate situation, he confronts the only remaining matter of importance—his concern about his center and the pain within his failing heart. With this failing center, he clearly sees how he has neglected the matters of his own heart. It is now time to recognize this failure and, at the same time, the achiever is forced to renounce all worldly things, as he finds he must confront his fear of death, dying, and departing. The question of "what remains?" arises. His dire situation casts out everything that is unimportant from his previous, hectic routine—an overly stimulated existence oriented towards the external life. As a mirror to the events of the physical body, the patient will also encounter his center—the focus of his life—on an emotional level.

His next station (the intensive-care unit) will help him to understand the gravity of his situation as the world of machinery and sophisticated survival technology becomes his reminder. The machines make him conscious of his heartbeat and force him to listen to it. They incessantly monitor his vital functions and scream a loud alarm if his heart deviates from a healthy pattern. He is connected to hoses; he is cabled with all these scientific devices; he is reduced to his vital functions; he practically becomes a part of the machine. The patient may, and should, become aware of how much he has tended to direct all of his attention to being a properly functioning person. He fulfilled his obligations as if he were a machine—reliable, orderly, calculating, and heartless. Has he not voluntarily reduced his life to a robot-like existence as it is now the case for his physical situation? It is now important to examine and accept what is dead and machinelike within oneself. After he has survived the heart attack, the person will encounter the principle of Saturn—here the planet is seen in a far more relentless form than its presentation to the angina-pectoris patient. The patient's entire "remaining life" now consists exclusively of concentrating on one thing—his heart—his center. He must now learn to concentrate on the essentials and limit his scope. He may have previously jumped through life like a sack of fleas and rushed from one obligation to the next challenge but now there is only one duty—he must concentrate on his own center, find his focus, and let everything that is superfluous fall away. The question of priorities in one's life may arise. Stimulated by the heart's rhythm problems, the patient raises health to the rank of necessity and his approach to life becomes more conscious. The theme of a tolerable rhythm in life may also arise. The forced rest that the heart induces the patient to take will also make the need for inner peace tangible.

In the meantime, the external situation has made it clear to everyone in the environment how the patient has fought with valor, with his back to the wall. At best, he can now admit this to himself. In the acute fear of losing his life, he could recognize his basic fear of losing himself. This deep fear requires the invoking of all the ego's boundary-setting and security measures. It is also this fear that has made him so constricted and closed off to other people. The senselessness of all of his grandiose activity can now become clear and understandable as a vain attempt to distract his mind from his insecurity. Setting boundaries only makes sense when something needs to be limited. However, as long as one's own core remains insecure, all meaning has gone. A person who depends on external factors and other people for validation has an arbitrary point of reference. As long as outside recognition and popularity with others are the central concerns, there is no personal center. The central station is everywhere and, therefore, it is nowhere at all. A person must first establish a life anchor; one must recognize and secure one's own center. Then, a purposefulness aimed towards a decisive point—the true goal of one's own life—can develop out of the patient's striving to "get ahead" at any price. The constricting sense of duty regarding countless obligations can evolve and it can become the resolved form—the patient's voluntary surrender to a higher responsibility. Unresolved ambitions of needing to be superior (no matter at what cost) can evolve into the perception that the greatest responsibility is to liberate one's own center. The patient must become familiar with his own heart and so he must learn to love himself and other people above all else. At this point, it has become clear that this incessant search for recognition—and the resulting addiction that comes from striving to reach goals through achievement—correspond, on the resolved level, with the deep longing to love and to be loved.

4.

The Embattled Heart

The general symptom known as inflammation occupies a central position in medical science. In earlier times, inflammations were even the main cause of death. Today, they are still by far the most frequent cause of illness. Medications have defused them to a considerable degree, but phlogistic states are still quite dangerous—not to mention the inconvenience that they cause. This is particularly appropriate when it involves a central organ such as the heart.

In the physical domain, inflammations tend to mimic the conditions of war and once more our idiomatic sentiments express this well. One speaks of an "inflammation *flare up"* or states that antibiotics are good *weapons* in the battle against pathogens. In general, one does not differentiate between the description of an emotional, martial, or inflammatory conflict. A political conflict is the incendiary spark for every military conflagration; in the same way, an igniting dispute precedes every war on the emotional level—every inflammation has its own triggering conflict.[9]

If one focuses on the significance of inflammations, one may recognize that even in our era the majority of the human race tends to live unconsciously when it comes to emotional conflict. A person who does not let himself be aroused by his personal conflict and does not even perceive it, lets the problem sink into the shadow and thereby opens up the body to pathogens. *Every infection is an embodied conflict.* The site of the occurrence shows symbolically the specific conflict theme through its physical manifestation. Inflammations in the area of the heart are consequently a central conflict, an unconscious battle for one's own physical center, one's own core, the center of life. However, the person has not consciously recognized this highly explosive situation and so the body becomes the substitute stage for the drama. As in all of these cases, it would be much easier if the conflict at hand had not shifted to another level in terms of time and space. A better motto would be: "Do not avoid any conflict!" However the fact that it occurs time and again is understandable. The original conflict must seem frightening to the soul, just as the substituting inflammation is a frightening experience for the body when it eventually manifests. The dangerous nature of heart inflammations, in turn, shows how threatening the primary conflicts are.

The course of inflammatory confrontation can erupt on the physical, emotional, and even on a national level. The shift from one level to another is also quite possible, although the step from an individual soul's conflict to an entire nation's conflict may seem quite large. Just as nations can end the battle at short notice in order to continue the fight at the negotiation table, a patient can suspend the war that has broken out in his body and continue it on the emotional level. However, the situation can reverse itself when the conditions become too confusing or when negotiations have failed. Then the struggle resumes once more on the battlefield. Whether the conflicts find expression with arguments, guns, or antibodies, the principle is identical. Once again, the choice lies between the conscious and the unconscious levels.

4.1 Rheumatic Carditis and Other Forms of Heart Inflammation

Because of its frequency and critical nature, rheumatic carditis holds a primary position among the inflammatory heart disorders. It can attack the heart muscle as *myocarditis,* the endocardium as *endocarditis,* and the pericardium as *pericarditis.* A streptococci infection must precede each of the three individual manifestations, which may even manifest at the same time. Streptococci are a type of bacteria distinguished by a very large number of different varieties and subgroups. They almost always initiate the inflammations that are the potential precursors of carditis: tonsillitis, sore throat, scarlet fever, erysipelas, and so-called latent infections. A lack of any acute stage from the onset of the disease and the absence of intense symptoms distinguish the latter category. Two to five weeks pass following these infections before any so-called rheumatic fever manifests itself. In medical terms, this is an allergic reaction of the body to parts of the streptococci, the antigens, that have settled in the heart and/or the joints. They can also help set the stage for the clinical syndrome of *glomerulonephritis* (kidney inflammation).

Therefore, the entire problem started with a conflict that did not succeed in creating space for itself within the patient's consciousness. However, on the physical level, the patient can no longer stop it from occupying the space denied to it on the level of consciousness. He must now let himself be shaken by the pathogens. The point that they attack depends on two factors that only seem to be different. First, the attacking point must offer the symbolically appropriate stage on which to perform the didactic play and second, the point must be a *locus minoris resistentiae,* (a weak spot) so the attack can be successful. In reality, the fulfillment of both of these requirements occurs at the same time—every conflict has a natural relationship to that part in the physical body to which it best corresponds. Even the refusal to create space for the conflict within the conscious mind prepares the appropriate substitute body part in that it makes it receptive as the mediator of the lesson. Yet, every opening to the outside automatically demands a weakening of the body's defenses. This permits the impending drama to commence immediately on the appropriate stage.

Therefore, the pathogens form their first bridgehead in the lymphatic defensive organs that protect the throat (the main entrance to the body) or they attack the skin (the border fortification against the outside world); there the pathogens try to settle. In long and energy-dissipating battles, the body's defense system succeeds in gaining control of the attackers by using all of the weapons available to it. In the process, even the general mobilization of fever is necessary; it is not possible to contain the conflict at a local level. The entire body has to challenge the invader. However, while the patient feverishly anticipates the solution to this difficult conflict (already anticipating that he will be the victor) the invaders prepare a treacherous retreat.

The legend of the Trojan War describes the appropriate archetype. The retreating invaders leave behind a present that seems to be harmless (in this case the remains of the defeated streptococci correspond to the Trojan Horse). Within a few weeks, these remains of war will provoke an immensely exaggerated reaction of the body; this poses a greater danger than the entire original attack. The body manifests a distinctly allergic reaction to these remains. The defenders can ascribe the blame for this dramatic experience wholly to themselves and their exaggerated defense.

There is definitely a good reason for this reaction (which is analogous to the story of the Trojan War). It has its correlations on the emotional level in that a person may have seemingly resolved certain conflicting emotions. However, if even slightly reminded of the controversial topic, this person's emotions may explode anew with unimaginable violence. A seemingly harmless conversation can have a liberal sprinkling of these little reminders in a completely innocuous manner. Only the relatively arbitrary association of the person's ideas and flights of fantasy would transform those reminders into such highly explosive emotional mines. People who unconsciously become victims of this interplay naturally tend to prepare their bodies for the corresponding experience they are going to create.

An allergy is a defensive process.[10] However, its danger never lies in the invaders, but always in the exaggerated and often life-threatening reaction of one's own defense system. The invaders are usually very harmless, such as pollen, grass seed, cat hair, household dust, or even the residue of long-defused bacteria. The immune system perceives itself to be under severe attack and so it immediately screams for general mobilization which results in what can be described as the symbolic transference of the respective invader. For the typical allergens listed above, a sexual meaning might be significant. As a type of seed, pollen is ultimately a symbol of insemination. Cat hair is reminiscent of the pussy cat and the corresponding theme, and people with allergies often regard sexual topics as unclean, and thus it bears an association with innocuous household dust.

Therefore, one might assume that it must be the inherent symbolic meaning of streptococci antigens that infuriates the defensive system so excessively. The secret denotation of these allergens is probably that they have managed to penetrate the body and settle themselves inside of it.

One can observe a similar purely emotional but nevertheless allergic reaction when middle-class patients learn that they or their children have lice or fleas. This is a fairly harmless situation, yet it sets the stage for an emotional uprising that resembles the immune system's response to an allergy.

The thought that something foreign has violated one's boundaries—even broken through them and practically made itself at home in one's most intimate parts seems to be a horrible thought for the afflicted person. However, these individuals are usually unconscious of their emotions in the acute situation—comparable to a rheumatic fever shuddering through the body. However, the defense system recognizes with horror the appalling invaders in the heart, kidneys, and joints. All of these three body parts symbolize areas that are both vulnerable and intimate: the joint cavities denote the basis for our flexibility, the kidneys represent our themes of partnership, and the heart symbolizes the center and focus of our existence.

The streptococci do not particularly threaten these sensitive zones in the physical sense, but the threat is all the more intense on the symbolic level. Characteristically, the defense system does not even attack right away. Instead, it leaves itself the two to five weeks that it uses to properly arm itself and to practice (metaphorically) shooting at the invaders, whom the defense system had already located long ago. Once the defensive system has become fully armed with precisely designed antibodies, it attacks without mercy. The damage does not occur so much through the battle, since the antigens are not at all capable of resistance; the physical harm occurs because of the unleashing of the colossal war machinery itself. One can compare this situation to a modern army; millions of troops use all of their war weapons to attack a tribe of practically unarmed Indians in the Amazon. The Indians have no defense with which to resist, yet the battlefield will become a tenable ruin.

The same thing happens to the heart in an attack of rheumatic fever. The concentrated power of the attack of the body overruns the streptococci antigens—no matter where they have concealed themselves. Not a single one can escape its fate, because the accuracy of the weapons developed by the immune system is overpowering. While the wave of attack rolls, the heart gets caught in an extremely threatening situation.

If the antigens travel to the muscle tissue, the heart begins to race and beats in a state of panic, called the *gallop rhythm*. The tissue fluid that collects during the inflammatory process can lead to edema between the individual muscle cells and thereby soften the structure of the heart to a certain degree. One possible consequence is the acute enlargement of the heart with a resulting relative mitral regurgitation. This means that the atrioventricular valve between the left atrium and ventricle can no longer close. As a result, the work of the heart becomes highly inefficient. In the process, the patient may develop a state of heart regurgitation. Ultimately, atrial flutter and fibrillation may occur. If this spreads to the ventricles of the heart, the end draws near. Even if things do not go this far, the entire heart falls to pieces.

If this affects the heart sac, the patient often experiences a massive *burning* pain in the chest. The medical profession calls such inflammations of the heart sac *pericarditis*. If such an inflammation-caused discharge appears in the heart sac, it can turn into a cardiac tamponade. In its lighter form, this can obstruct the heart; however, if it reaches considerable dimensions, it can even strangle it. The most dangerous complication of the remitting heart-sac discharge is the incomplete reabsorption of the materials contained in the fluid, such as protein, white and red blood cells, and coagulation-promoting fibrin. Above all, fibrin can gather into a mass and settle in the heart which is the condition that has led to the diagnostic expression *hairy heart*. If the situation has an even less favorable outcome, solid scar tissue forms in the cleft of the heart sac and this can grow deeply into the muscle tissue and frequently even *calcify*. In this case, the medical diagnostic term is *armor heart*. However, if it is a dry form of pericarditis, the characteristic noises of friction accompany every movement of the heart.

If antigens have settled on the inner lining of the heart, endocarditis occurs. Frequently associated with it is the fearsome valvular defect. More than half of all children and up to one-third of adults—who suffer from the above symptoms—develop such valvular defects. These defects mainly occur in the area of the left heart (for instance, in the mitral and aortic valve). In the process, the endocarditis usually begins quite mildly; sometimes it can even be completely overlooked and misdiagnosed as severe arthritic pain. However, the previous battle has left traces on the pericardium that become obvious in due course. As a result of the rheumatic fever, small wart-like deposits form mainly on the cusps of the heart valves and their tendon fibers; this causes no symptoms apart from slight flowing sounds. The edematous swelling also creates no problems. The actual defects occur through the scarring of the battle traces on the pericardium. On the one hand, the scarred shrinking of the valve cusps and the tendon fibers that hold them can lead to the constriction of the circulatory pathway (stenosis). On the other hand, it can bring about the valve's inability to close (regurgitation). In both cases, the work of the heart can experience considerable impediments depending on the extent of the defect. In the case of stenosis, the valve suddenly obstructs the blood flow, mimicking that of river rapids. The heart must create more pressure in order to press the same amount of blood through the bottleneck. The blood swirls around, giving rise to the danger of clot formation. In the case of regurgitation, the valve closes incompletely and it more or less loses its function as a valve. The blood that flows in the reverse direction disrupts the work of the heart and, most importantly, ruins its effectiveness. The next chapter describes valvular defects in considerable detail.

The prognosis differs greatly for the various cases of endocarditis. This is a good thing in the case of slight defects which have little effect on life expectancy. In comparison, severe valvular defects are very serious; they can even lead to death through embolism or cardiac regurgitation. After the initial episode, others usually follow, resulting in the worsening state of the heart defect.

Naturally, the meaning of heart-inflammation symptoms for the patient depends to a great degree on their severity. Behind the most impressive form of myocarditis which causes the entire heart to fall to pieces there is a heart-ache of such magnitude that it could turn a normal life upside down. One may say that this conflict actually places one's life at stake. Understandably, the affected person prefers to avoid such a confrontation. However, it is no less dangerous when it transfers onto the physical heart. In the physical case, the patient feels that it is a matter of life or death. A war that is both painful and bitter has flared up for the heart. Because of the unconscious nature of the painful emotional aspect, the patient has unintentionally chosen the painful physical path. The pain in her chest gives her the impression that her heart is on fire. Her heart is aflame in an emotional sense and the situation is so rife with conflict that she prefers to shut her eyes to it. As a consequence, she must now experience the battle—that she did not want to fight—being fought by her physical heart with every fiber of this organ. In the process, the heart apparently begins to weep inwardly; the tears penetrate between its cells and soften the solid structure. As a result, the heart enlarges under the pressure of its own actions and in many cases, its valves will no longer completely close.

Once again, it becomes particularly clear that processing the energy of this conflict on the emotional level would have been much more tolerable than having to deal with its life-endangering incarnation in the physical heart. If only the patient had cried her heart out early enough, and had her heart broadened or—at least—allowed a softer attitude to relax her strictly closed emotions; her tragic feelings might still have threatened the structure of her life, but they would not have threatened her physical survival. If one would like to extend the symbolic parallels even further, one might say, "The old Adam must die," in either the figurative sense or in very concrete terms.

The other individual symptoms listed above substantiate and vary this basic theme. The racing heart and the gallop rhythm are expressions of the panic that the conflict has triggered in the patient and, at the same time, also reflect its tendency. Racing can be alluded to as a type of swift escape velocity. A person usually attempts to race away when he feels himself threatened on an existential level and this clearly applies to the victim in terms of both the emotional heart conflict and the physical cardiac inflammation. The gallop is the way that horses take if they want to escape and the heartbeat imitates this behavior in panic situations. We have already investigated heart flutter and fibrillation in the similar situation of a heart attack, the heart's breaking down at the death's door, when it has exhausted its reserves, when discomfort has overstepped intolerable levels.

In its acute stage, pericarditis also reveals a conflicting theme that smolders (in the truest sense of the word) in the heart of the afflicted person. Yet, it does not affect the muscles but is limited to its outer skin. In this case, the tears of the heart force their way to the outside. These are not very dangerous if there are not too many of them. However, the heart can drown in them if they greatly increase, or one does not appease them in time. If we remain with the allegorical description, the chronic stages of pericarditis command respect; the condition called *hairy heart* resembles a fragile object that is packed in tissue, while *armor heart* seems to be embedded in marble. Marble is composed mainly of calcium which is an absolutely inappropriate protective material. Therefore, the afflicted person has essentially set up a tombstone in the middle of his own heart. The inscription on it tells of a cruel history, namely, the poor treatment that the heart has suffered, despite the fact (or precisely because of it) that the owner tried to protect it and shield it from everything. There is also enough evidence through its many scars, that it has petrified itself into its scarred armor. A person suffering from *hairy heart* is forcing his physical heart to embody the theme of an overly insulated psyche; in the figurative sense, he is trying to protect the heart from everything and in effect has wrapped it in tissue. All of the emotional conflicts of the heart (that the consciousness has tried to spare itself) have left behind their wounds and the scars that resulted from them. The danger from exaggerated protection finds a very clear representation in the extremely breakable *armor heart* that, instead of presenting an image of security, tends to convey the impression of paralysis. The person who wants to spare himself of everything will not be spared of anything. "He who would save his life shall lose it."

The opposite extreme of openness and expansiveness is, naturally, the salvation that comes from facing this situation of being armored to death. Despite this, the patient must admit that his primary concern is the protection of his heart—his center. The course of the disorder shows him this task very clearly; he has turned the heart into a fortress that is invincible from the outside. Consequently, more solidity of the heart and firmness on the emotional level is necessary. The task is to learn to defend one's own center and to consciously build a solid fortress that provides enough protection and security. A person must also learn to close off his territorial boundaries if he does not want to lose himself completely. From this secure position (one's own center) one can risk steps to reach the opposite pole. Before one can do this, the important themes seem to be limitation and wise restriction, concentrating on what is essential, and—in extreme cases—reconciliation with the last and most fundamental theme—death.

In contrast, the story behind dry heart-sac inflammation tends to be quite dry itself. No tears flow, but it becomes clear that the movements within one's own center no longer function without friction. Instead, they give the impression of an unlubricated machine struggling in its last motions. Doctors have named these noises *to-and-fro sounds,* probably because the sonification reminded them of the chugging sound of an old locomotive. Apparently, the person is not having an easy time dealing with the conflicts that revolve around his own center. Things no longer run smoothly, but sluggishly and laboriously. The conflicts that have undergone the suppression process are probably just as tough and grueling. If the individual had faced them, these feelings of strife would probably also have "taken the grease out of the machinery" of life for some time, and coping with existence would have been more difficult. However, the spiritual-emotional conflict level remains the only one with genuine prospects for a solution.

In addition to the rheumatic forms of heart inflammation, there are several other forms of inflammation that employ different pathogens and different origins. For example, there is a form of myocarditis that follows diphtheria, occurring directly in the muscle cells and not in the interstices (interstitial tissue). Another variation is influenzal myocarditis that usually runs a very benign course and, at most, it becomes conspicuous because of the so-called *extrasystoles.* These also occur on many other occasions; and they may be interpreted as a kind of "stumbling" of the heart. When a person stumbles while he walks, it shows that he has minor problems with alertness on the path that he is taking; the same principle applies to extrasystoles. The heart demands a bit more attention and gets it through its stumbling pace. Furthermore, there are a series of infectious diseases that may accompany an inflammation of the cardiac muscle. However, in essence, the symptoms and therefore their meaning are not different from those that this book has already outlined.

The majority of the clinical syndromes that encourage the two other forms of heart inflammation can also promote a pericarditis. They frequently occur as an accompanying symptom of a heart attack. In addition to the important rheumatic pericarditis, the tubercular and idiopathic forms are particular examples. *Idiopathic* means self-suffering; this is just another way of implying that medical science does not know what has caused the inflammation. However, since all of these forms develop comparable symptoms, they also lead to similar interpretations.

In addition to the streptococci antigens, an endocarditis can trigger a whole series of pathogens by settling on the endocardium (the inner skin of the heart). In particular, they settle in the cusp valves and tendon fibers. In the long term, they can lead to ulcerous changes, purulent tissue liquefactions, clot formation, and valve defects. A high fever usually brings the corresponding conflict to a boil; vehement chills shake the patient.

Endocarditis lenta is a long-lasting inflammation of the inner heart skin without these acute symptoms; however, it does result in the same valve defect. In this case, these are essentially harmless germs that actually even form a part of normal skin and mucous-membrane flora. They normally show little aggression but will assail a previously damaged heart, in the manner of the proverb "opportunity makes the thief." The interpretation of this process deviates from the other forms—the person should admit that her own center has already suffered severe damage and weakening. Very harmless conflicts—usually innocuous during normal conditions—can be sufficiently serious to threaten the heart and cause severe defects and obstructions. We will take a closer look at the meaning of these later. The whole process takes place in such a slow and sneaky manner that it hardly attracts any attention for a long period of time.

4.2 The Weapons of Orthodox Medicine

A single word can summarize the popular therapy employed by orthodox medicine for practically all forms of heart inflammations: antibiotic—meaning *against life!* This naturally is supposed to threaten the lives of the intruders and attackers. Antibiotics are genuinely sophisticated weapons aimed at the vital functions of bacteria to inactivate them. The best-known antibiotic is penicillin, which is a very popular weapon in the battle against the pathogens of heart inflammations; it is a product from the mold *Aspergillus penicillinum*. This is a genuine natural remedy. The offensive bacteria mistake the penicillin molecule for a building substance that is important for their wall structure; so the invaders erroneously incorporate it into themselves. When the new bacteria has finished their construction work, the penicillin suddenly no longer keeps its promise as a building substance, and the newly completed young bacteria dies.

This warfare is somewhat insidious, since its success relies on false promises and crass deception; it is highly successful in the acute inflammatory stage. With this technique, medical science provides the body with a virtual mercenary troop that effectively supports its struggle for defense. The foundation for the strategy of the enemy bacteria rests on the working army's production through tremendous reproductive activity after it has established a bridgehead in the body. The original invasion army is of secondary significance in terms of numbers, and if it were dependent on only itself, it could never become dangerous. The body's own defensive troops would very quickly eradicate these first invaders. Through the antibiotics, the bacteria experience obstruction from carrying out this decisive act of their own reproduction. They can neither recruit new troops nor replace their comrades in arms which have fallen in the battle of the body's defenses.

In this hopeless situation, they either give up or shift to another battle strategy. Since antibiotics reach bacteria solely through the blood stream, they can *dig in* somewhere else away from it. When they have *entrenched* themselves, a situation similar to typical trench warfare begins. In such a war of position (such as at the end of the World War I), both sides can exhaust their forces and, without victory on either side, the conflict becomes chronic. This is one of the sources of danger for heart inflammations. Despite antibiotic support, relative strength can remain balanced. This occurs either because a person's own defensive power is so weak or because the invader has so cleverly chosen its position. In the case of the heart, they sit in the middle of a person's center like in a fortress.

One of the disadvantages of the antibiotic auxiliary troops now becomes evident. The indiscriminate use of antibiotics at every opportunity can be self-defeating; the body starts to depend on them and becomes increasingly incapable of defending itself. Similarly, a country that constantly relies on outside help will also gradually become dependent on that help because its own armed forces no longer receive training. This situation is particularly fatal when the attacker resorts to a second tactic. After having fallen for the trick of false building blocks for a long enough time, one bacterium will eventually become smart enough to adapt and it will modify its behavior according to this wretched state of affairs. For example, if it finds a minor alteration in the wall, it now has enormous developmental advantages because it can merrily continue to reproduce while its conservative comrades suffer annihilation by the millions. In the not too distant future, the entire bacteria army will consist of its next generation. Unobstructed by the antibiotics, they will all be able to reproduce. This demonstrates the second dangerous disadvantage of the antibiotics, because they contribute considerably to the breeding of new strains of bacteria which are even more dangerous because they are less vulnerable.

Medical science then speaks of the development of resistance. The prospects may seem optimistic for the practice of antibiotic therapy on acute inflammations; however, the situation is just as dismal for the chronic case. Unfortunately, heart inflammations are no exception in that regard.

In addition, orthodox medicine uses the drug cortisone for particularly severe cases of infection when the danger of hazardous scar formation exists. In essence, this is also a natural remedy; cortisone is a hormone produced by the adrenal cortex within one's own body. Cortisone is one of the body's most effective stress hormones; cortisone production occurs primarily in situations concerning pure survival. It mobilizes all of the necessary energies for lifesaving purposes while setting aside the immunological defense processes. It even stops the defenses from becoming active.

One might say that cortisone is an antidote for the body— that its purpose is to protect the body from acting out what the conscious mind should be processing but is not. In the case of a heart inflammation, cortisone also prevents the body from portraying the conflict-laden drama that has just broken out around the heart. It also prohibits the body from setting the stage. However, the conflict must have a field of expression somewhere. The useful measure is to bring it back to the level of consciousness, requiring a great deal of emotional openness. Cortisone can even promote such feeling in this case, however, doctors usually employ this remedy with the opposite intention. The patient did not want to confront the originating conflict on the level of consciousness and therefore suppressed it; now he is also trying to avoid confrontation on the physical level while at the same time suppressing the emotions. Antibiotics are used with similar intentions.

But the conflict must expose itself somewhere in the physical body. It must have some projective surface conceded to it. If neither the soul nor the body tolerate it, it will project itself outside the individual into the social realm and in this case it will take the form of conflicts—naturally, as dispute and war. Despite

The Embattled Heart

our hatred of conflict, it is no coincidence that crises and small wars shake our world. The projection continues vigorously on this level and one can well observe this since both sides always feel completely justified—in the political as well as the personal dimension. Wars are almost always the planned products of secretaries of *defense,* but hardly ever, secretaries of *war.* In contrast, the word *armed forces* is refreshingly honest.

If a person is successful in projecting the battle of his own heart out of his body into the social environment, he should prepare for certain events to happen. The original conflicts ultimately are directed at the victim's spiritual center; the enemy pathogens are aimed for the victim's heart. Consequently, the external enemies that must now assume their function are more than just cardboard figures, and they will give their full effort to hit their target.

The suppressive intentions of orthodox medical therapy becomes quite clear through the so-called antiphlogistic (anti-inflammatory) agents in the line of treatments such as salicylic acid which one also uses for heart inflammations (for example, aspirin—acetylsalicylic acid). Translated to the emotional level, this corresponds to an agent that inhibits conflicts. Good examples of this could be plugging the ears or taping the mouth shut. These examples may be somewhat ludicrous, but they are no more misleading than the corresponding medical examples. In this manner, one can definitely inhibit the acting out of conflicts but the conflicts themselves apparently are inevitable. Neither salicylic acid nor cortisone are able to do any more than this.

The fourth weapon of orthodox medicine is the family of painkillers and morphine holds the first position in this group. This book has already mentioned its great value and the suppressive nature of this drug is quite obvious. Yet, when the heart screams so intensely for help that the patient can no longer bear these screams, the best and only appropriate action is to relieve the perception of pain through morphine. The danger of painfully plugging someone's ears so that they cannot hear warning signals is the allegory for the special case of morphine, but it hardly bears mentioning. There is an addictive syndrome to consider and there is principally no difference between long-term morphine therapy and carrying on a long-term (albeit, necessary) suppressive medication for acute lifesaving measures.

Another special therapy is the aspiration of the heart sac in order to drain fluid and, thereby, intervene in pericarditis with fluid in the heart sac. This measure can prevent the life-threatening tamponade. However, even this convincing reason presents the danger of habituation occurring. If the surgeon suctions the discharge fluid too frequently, the body lends to continue to produce the discharge as it needs this expression to represent its theme of conflict. In the same way that a farmer can stimulate a cow's udder to produce more milk by persistently milking it, one can also train a heart to constantly secrete fluid. This lead to the image of the continuously weeping heart, a condition which results in a considerable loss of protein for the body at a time when the organism cannot afford this depletion.

By now, we have almost found an answer to the question of how to relieve the clinical pictures presented so far. Instead of continuously suppressing conflicts, it makes far more sense to face them and solve them on the conscious level.

Whenever inflammations are noticeable in the body, it is best for a person to admit that his conflicts have, once again, slipped back down to the physical level. It would be best if the person identifies the inflammatory productions on the physical stage through the emotional conflict. When a person has located this, it is a matter of living out the conflict and confronting it—letting the sparks fly on this level, instead of permitting the heart to fall to pieces.

It will not always be possible to act out a conflict and thereby resolve it. Even after the hottest discussions and the most vehement *battles* of words, the separating trenches may remain deep. Sometimes a verbal duel can even increase the aggressive pressure on the opponents during the confrontation. All of this is comparatively harmless as long as the conflict remains in the conscious mind and does not become suppressed. If a

The Embattled Heart

person succeeds in consciously tolerating the unbreachable tension, there is no danger that the theme will slip down into the body as an inflammation. This only happens if a person pretends to reconcile for the sake of peace in a situation that is truly irreconcilable. The body corrects such insincerity with the use of its theatrics by demonstrating what is really happening. However, the honest conflict, the acute emotional dissatisfaction, the most vehement quarrel, and even a violent altercation are naturally no reason to stage an incendiary drama. As long as the topic still smolders in the heart in the figurative sense, and flaming volleys are being shot back and forth, the physical heart will not go up in flames. On the contrary, the heart will pump for all it is worth in order to provide its owner with the necessary energy for the aggressive confrontation. Also, the pumping will be unbelievably good and the heart will keep working for a long time because it is in its element when it churns. A great deal has to happen before it runs into difficulties while fulfilling this task. However, its threshold of pain approaches more quickly on the much less appropriate level of expressing emotional dramas. As long as the tears of anger and pain still flow from the eyes, they will not flood into the tissue as inflammatory exudate; the heat of the confrontation will virtually protect the corresponding tissue from inflammatory overheating.

In this case, the leap into the opposite pole quickly and obviously reveals itself to be a flight. Peace and quiet may also become the goal at some point, but initially this is a matter of battle. Although peace and quiet may represent higher values, they remain inappropriate and, therefore, one should not even expect to achieve them in the long term if they are uncalled for at the moment. In the short term, the offer of peace gains time in the acute situation when one has bridged the great gulf on one level. This is how orthodox medicine with its intense use of antibiotics, cortisone, anti-phlogistics, and painkillers achieves a brief and welcome breather but not more. With this ride at full speed on the four allopathic horses, we reach the opposite pole of repose and relaxation; however, it is not possible to maintain this state by the same means. If we do not metaphorically re-saddle and put our faith in other horses, the inflammation will flare up again.

Aggression, that ultimately stands behind all conflicts and confrontations, is a fundamental force of our existence. It is certain that we will never be able to settle all the problems with it; this is probably lucky for us as well. Even if we give it our complete effort, we will probably suffer from inflammations, and re-experience the aggression that has only been slightly redressed. The Bhagavad Gita, a central work of India's holy writings, outlines precisely this theme in a conversation between the warrior Arjuna and the god Krishna. The noble fighter Arjuna wants to renounce an armed conflict, with the loftiest of intentions, but the god Krishna sends him into the battle.

5.

The Defective Heart

5.1. Congenital Heart Defects and Responsibility

On the physical level, one can subdivide the defects of the heart into two groups—acquired (such as consecutive symptoms of rheumatic fever) and congenital. The latter pose some intellectual problems, since the Western world tends to absolve the newborn child of any responsibility for its newly begun existence. A person from the Eastern traditions does not have this kind of difficulty when it comes to appropriately interpreting the congenital symptoms of adult illness. Eastern philosophy assumes reincarnation to be a fact with as much conviction as many religions in the West challenge it.

Those who believe in many earthly lives naturally have little problem in understanding congenital symptoms; these they recognize as learning tasks that the infant has brought along into this life. It cannot be the task of this book to formulate any judgment on a topic such as reincarnation, but a certain openness to the idea would be quite advantageous. In this sense, an unprejudiced viewpoint can help in analyzing the circumstantial facts. These show that a negative attitude towards reincarnation represents a minority opinion throughout the entire world. This statement naturally does not prove anything, but it nevertheless clarifies the proportional relationship.

To date, it has not been possible to disprove the idea of reincarnation scientifically, and it will not be possible in the future. On the other hand, there are now an abundance of well-proven examples of rebirth. Above all, the American neurologist and psychiatrist, Ian Stevenson,[11] has collected and documented hundreds of such cases. A great deal of practical experience with reincarnation therapy has ultimately resulted in many indications in this direction. Even in our Christian religion one can still find a belief in rebirth. An example of this appears in the story when the disciples ask Christ if He were the reborn Elijah. The belief in reincarnation was still present during the first Christian century; this is proven by statements of the early church fathers.

Regarding congenital defects, only pure desperation, or the projection of guilt on an unjust God (or an unjust fate) remains for those who cannot accept the perspective of reincarnation. What should one think of a God (or fate) that lets children grow up well formed and healthy in wonderful parental homes, while permitting others to be deformed and live a miserable existence in poverty and without parents? As hard as it already may be to place the burden of responsibility for its destiny on a newborn child, the alternative of assuming that God is unjust is probably even more deplorable.

The experiences of reincarnation therapy can reveal that behind every symptom there is a learning task. Also, the organization of the Creation is by far not as unjust as it may seem to our short-sighted perspective restricted to the opinion of a singular lifetime.[12]- There is a message in every symptom; therefore, it is an opportunity that fate has offered. Every clinical picture illustrates a symbolic path that the patient takes either consciously or unconsciously and that offers him the opportunity to reach his goal.

5.2 Various Congenital Heart Defects

Defective developments of the heart and its large vessels manifest themselves in great variety and they are extremely complicated. However, the most important forms are based on an incorrect or incomplete adaptation of the embryonic cardiovascular system. In its embryonic development, the human being once again virtually follows the path of life, leading from the primeval sea to solid land. During the early period in the amniotic fluid, the placenta is the organ that supplies the circulation of oxygen. It is neither possible nor necessary for the embryo to breathe on its own. With birth into the airy world of polarity, breathing becomes compulsory. The lobes of the lung, which have been folded up to this point, must now unfurl. They do this with the first breath or cry of the newborn baby. Because of the changed pressure condition, the *ductus arteriosus*—the blood vessel that had previously guided the venous blood into the aorta by circumventing the heart—closes reflexively. At the same time, the septum of the heart closes and the one large heart chamber transforms into two, in order to meet the tasks of life in the polarized world—the world of opposites.

For the newborn child, this adaptation is probably about as difficult as the corresponding step that sea animals made to solid land eons ago. It can happen that the complete adaptation does not occur; and individual relics from the early epoch remain. Holding on to what has been well-proven becomes an obstacle for life, since it is no longer appropriate for the new situation. In this case, medical science speaks of a *congenital heart defect*.

5.2.1 Defects of the Heart Septum

For defects of the heart septum, physical unity of the heart is more or less retained. In the extreme case, the affected children remain closer to unity than to life within polarity and to their bodies. The hole in the heart, called a *septal defect* in medical terms, can lie in the atrium or the ventricle region. Since the pressure during the contraction phase of the heart is considerably higher on the left side, a short circuit occurs and the oxygen-rich blood of the left side flows to the right side. The pressure is about four times higher in the left ventricle than it is in the right ventricle; a large hole in the septum would cause a correspondingly large volume of blood to desert and change sides. Medical doctors then speak of a *left-right shunt*. Because the flow resistance is much too low in the pulmonary circulation, the lung overflows with four to five times the amount of blood that it requires. Many children die during this phase—during the first weeks of their lives. These deaths still occur even today, in the age of highly sophisticated heart surgery.

In those who survive, the vessels of the pulmonary circulation become accustomed to the additional stress as they adapt to it by thickening their walls. The pressure conditions adjust to those of the left side, and a balance becomes established so that no more shunt blood results and the pulmonary congestion eventually subsides. However, an arteriosclerosis develops in the lung vessels; the permanently increased pressure causes the resistance to increase even further, which gives rise to this condition. The pressure on the right side ultimately even exceeds that of the left side and the shunt reverses direction. Depending upon the extent of the disorder, this phase occurs between the first and tenth year of life. At this point, the low-oxygen blood from the right heart reaches the left side and from there, the systematic circulation results in a blue coloring of the skin. These children are handicapped in their development and limited in their functional capacity from the start. In addition to shortness of breath—due to the initial inundations—frequent infections in the lung area occur.

With this impressive clinical picture, the body displays an apparent state of being suspended in an early stage of development and one is inclined to imagine that it wants to retain the condition of *Unity*—the state of Paradise—in the womb. It seems to prefer to remain devoid of all responsibility and worry. This also manifests in the later behavior of the children who usually

The Defective Heart

feel compelled to hang onto their parental "apron strings" because they are not strong enough to withstand stress and are susceptible to infections. The problems with breathing reflect their continued difficulties in adapting to the world of polarity. The opposite principles of inhaling and exhaling, dependent as they are on each other, symbolize with particular distinction how much a person is at the mercy of the world of opposites. As long as one lives, one must succumb to the interplay of the breathing principle. Chronic infections in the lungs indicate how conflict-oriented this area is for the patient. Although the lobes of the lungs have unfolded, their owner is not really ready to stand on his own feet. The primeval sea that he has just left is now practically imitated by his lungs. Where air should be, water collects and the body demonstrates the tendency to regress by this action. This is precisely what the patient's every expression is leading up to. Instead of warming up to life and romping around in the world with rosy cheeks, these children communicate that they are perpetually on the verge of slipping away (by turning blue).

The clinical picture is very clear, but what benefit is this to a small child? It is not possible to start psychotherapy and he cannot find a solution by treating the principle of the problem intellectually or on a conscious level. At this point, it should be particularly clear that illness is a valid way to resolve a difficult theme. Every individual experiences and survives many colds in the course of his life—usually without achieving the slightest illumination regarding the particular theme to which one can no longer *warm up*. Instead, a person simply comes down with a cold or, as one may very insightfully put it, he "catches a cold." Going through this situation is apparently an adequate treatment for the suppressed theme so that the cold can disappear (the emotional energy can dissipate). The person with a cold has emphatically had a "nose full" and no longer wants to see or hear anything. He prefers to be completely alone, at best with a blanket over his head. However, this is exactly the theme that he must become aware of. The symptom brings it to consciousness—whether the person wants it or not.

In this respect, there is no reason to underestimate the ability of children to learn. They naturally learn in a different manner than adults and in many areas they are even better at learning because they apparently learn with more than just their heads. This is quite evident when learning a foreign language. Modern training methods place considerable emphasis on trying to simulate childlike learning in adults. This goal is achieved (e.g., in methods such as Superlearning) by more or less switching off the intellect.

Therapeutic experiences with children confirm their advantages for dealing with their own symptoms, and these advantages are similar to those they use when they learn a language. Children usually have a very good sense of what they are lacking from deep in their hearts. The moving experiences that Elizabeth Kübler-Ross[13] has had with dying children reveal this in a way that often brings humility to adults.

As long as their environment has not ruined them, children have a particularly good feeling for what they need and what is necessary when they are ill. When children catch a cold, they usually behave very cleverly. They do not eat—particularly if they are feverish—they drink a great deal, and *sleep themselves well.* Every sick animal acts in exactly the same way and regains its health as quickly as possible. In contrast, adults in comparable situations tend to maltreat their bodies with overly nutritious food; they sabotage the body's defenses with fever-sinking agents and usually they cannot afford the luxury of staying in bed. In reality, they are really preventing themselves from becoming healthy. This treatment also has its valid side, since adults generally need more time to work through the same theme. If they get healthy too quickly, they have to return to the same situation from which they have just fled.

Unfortunately, the situation is much more serious in the case of a heart defect but, luckily, the same principles function. The small patients experience their own drama more intensely with

The Defective Heart

body and soul; they learn astonishingly well from their handicapped situation. They display a lesser tendency to flee to the opposite extreme—much less than their parents. Naturally they long to romp around as if they were healthy children. However, most of them accept their destiny of being different—often better than their parents accept their fate of having a child that is so different.

The lessons to be learned are forcefully pushed through by the symptoms. Standing apart, during all physical activities and the most interesting games, creates an isolation which arises because the desire for some form of escape becomes very conscious. The desire to remain attached to the mother becomes painfully apparent in not being physically able to let her go. Romanticism in particular has tended to glorify the permanent closeness of such children to their Creator. In any case, a child in this situation becomes very conscious of how poor his chances are in this world because of his defective heart. Clinging to *Unity* has transmuted to the experience of loneliness and aloneness; when a child cannot keep up with his peers, he becomes the permanent outsider who remains in the distant background. Every form of being physically assertive and interactive is difficult for the child.

A flood of emotional themes dominate in the area of communication—so much so that conflicts constantly inflame the child as a result and these feelings show the child the enormity of his difficulties in the polarized world of the breath. This world of duality—that the child wanted to avoid—remains oddly strange and full of discord and despair. The child becomes the typical outsider, shut out from many things and thereby he experiences the implications of not opening up to the world. The tightly held theme of *Unity* remains, as it imposes itself upon the child in unresolved forms of loneliness and aloneness.

If one can believe the stories of the Romantic period or a tale such as Manfred Kyber's[14] *The Three Candles of Little Veronica,* it is sometimes possible to resolve such difficult situations. The experience of loneliness results in an all-oneness, of being everything in the whole. Serious illness then provides the great opportunity of mystically experiencing the world and, hence, the perception that it is not necessary—not even possible—to leave *Unity* because it eternally is everything; one always contains it within oneself.

The only possible medical therapy is surgical closing of the hole in the heart. However, this only promises success if it is performed before the shunt has reversed directions. Afterwards, the lungs are already so damaged that closing the defective septum no longer effects any improvement in the child's physical well being.

5.2.2 Problems with Old Paths

Another important congenital heart defect develops due to holding onto a structure that fulfilled a purpose before birth, but is very hindering after birth. It occurs when the ductus arteriosus—which guided the embryonic blood past the still folded fetal lungs—remains open. This condition is called *patent ductus arteriosus*. It was a very useful tool for diverting the blood before birth. However, this side street becomes a dangerous detour if it remains open instead of naturally atrophying and the blood truly gets on the wrong track. The proper direction of flow is reversed, and both sides of the heart are considerably overstrained. In the womb, blood flows from the right ventricle into the aorta and bypasses the lungs. However, after birth the pressure in the aorta is four times greater than the pulmonary circulation which reverses the direction of flow. The oxygen-rich blood of the aorta practically makes a U-turn and returns to the lungs. Immediately afterwards, it flows into the left heart.

One observes a similar situation when the septum is defective, but in this case the shunt lies outside the heart. As a result, the left side of the heart increases in strength because of the additional stress. The increased blood supply to the lungs and the higher pressure give rise to arteriosclerosis. The pressure in the pulmonary circulation ultimately increases, causing the shunt to stop and even reverse itself. Then it is too late for surgical correction. The embryonic situation has been recreated, blood lacking in oxygen reaches the circulatory system by detouring around the lungs, and the patient turns blue. Life in this world does not permit a circumvention of the principle of polarity and the lungs. Exchange and communication have become vital processes for life. If one does not subject oneself to the game of opposites in the lungs, one turns blue.

Even though the symptoms and signs are similar to those of the septum defects, the situation is by no means as acute. Frequently, during athletic activities the person first notices that he is not capable of exercising over a longer period of time and can quickly suffer from a pounding heart and shortness of breath. His carotid artery visibly displays the battle of the heart to other observers. The affected individuals are outwardly similar to the patients with aortic regurgitation because they look slightly strained and yet full of pulsating life. Typically, the patent ductus arteriosus is manifested in women than in men.

Through the symptom, it becomes emphatically clear to the patient that she is taking the false path with her vital energy. The blood that has gotten on the wrong track practically rotates more or less in vain, making it obvious that the fetal shortcut has now turned into a real-life detour, lacking any advantages whatsoever. Instead, the situation only brings considerable disadvantages. When this has become clear on all levels of depth, the surgeon can successfully eliminate the wrong pathway by tying up the vessel that has become superfluous.

5.2.3 Alarming Reminders of Old Times

The coarctation of the aorta also is a reminder of the previous ductus arteriosus. Although it has atrophied and turned into a tendinous band in this case, it constricts the aorta, particularly when the person is older. This constriction usually does not have an effect during childhood. When the aorta grows during adolescence, the narrow area remains unchanged and thereby turns into a circulatory obstruction. Since the old ductus arteriosus first started on the other side of the heart's exit to the upper-body supply vessels, the constriction keeps the supply to the upper body intact while the abdomen receives less and less blood. The heart must increase the blood pressure in order to send any blood down to it and so the typical signs of high blood pressure develop in the upper body while low blood pressure dominates the lower parts of the body. High blood pressure becomes noticeable in the upper body through the reddened face and pulsating carotid artery while, in the lower body, the feet are cold and no pulse can be felt. A further emergency measure that the body can lake is to construct bypasses that will divert a little additional blood down past the narrow areas.

The dangers of this clinical picture correspond to those of high blood pressure for the upper body. Arteriosclerosis, cardiac regurgitation, and the disposition toward strokes are particularly noteworthy. In addition, there is the imminent danger of a rupture in the aorta at the narrowed spot.

The symbolic meaning of these symptoms becomes more vivid in the following interpretation of high blood pressure and cardiac regurgitation. As always, the specific meaning of the coarctation of the aorta can be deduced from the symptoms. While the upper body is pulsating with life, the abdomen has been cut off from the supply of vital energy. Apparently, this reflects a drastic psychosomatic preference for the body's upper (masculine) portion to the detriment of the lower (feminine) part. The discrimination against the feminine portion goes so far that the lifelessness and fear with respect to this area becomes clear in the manifestation of perpetually cold feet. Sexuality is also obstructed since it depends on an abundance of blood in the genitalia. The person in question is completely closed to the lower feminine area of life and those themes associated with it, especially sexuality and procreation. The upper body reacts by closing itself off and in some cases it blocks its vessels extensively against the rush of blood. The problematical nature becomes even more critical because the legs feel the effects as does the lower torso. This, in turn, influences the development and progress of the person.

The temporal evolution of these symptoms clarifies the fear of the lower feminine area of life even more. They occur precisely at a developmental phase when it is important to integrate the organs of the abdomen with its themes into life. Instead, the development in the area of the aortic isthmus becomes retarded (this also includes the development of the abdomen). One can see how severe the fear and constriction are by the fact that some patients would prefer to allow the connection with their lower half to break off (rupture of the aorta) rather than provide it with sufficient vital energy. They would rather die than open themselves up to the problem at hand.

With these symptoms, the task is to become aware and cognizant of the negative attitude towards the lower feminine polarity in the first place. This is certainly not a fully conscious awareness, since the symptoms then would be unnecessary. Before a person can begin to resolve this theme (and, thereby, conquer the opposite pole), he must first consciously reconcile himself with the effective principles of constriction. This applies to the one-sided preference of the masculine area in particular. Concentration and limitation as more developed expressions of the principles of constriction and fear have already been presented a number of times. Directing them toward the theme of the upper body and the head (at masculinity and intellectuality) may open up new pathways. Instead of automatically endowing these areas with vital energy on the physical level, conscious mental energies should be directed against those areas as well. However, when these upper themes are consciously resolved, understanding and longing for the opposite pole occur quite naturally.

Those who energetically concentrate on the themes of the head and the masculine principle in the intellectual sense will at some point also need to have a physical basis for the perceptions of his mind. Among the primary masculine principles are activity and aggression, as well as penetration into new areas. Yet, the conscious resolution of such themes leads downwards towards the abdomen—to masculine sexuality—that relates to the penetration into new contrasting areas on the physical level.

A consciously experienced extreme of reality always demands the opposite pole for its resolution. Just as inhaling requires exhaling, the masculine longs for the feminine and vice versa. Even on the physical level, this compensating need of the body is apparent in the case of the vessels of the upper body which are lavished with energy. They eventually constrict and during a stroke an entire part of the brain is deprived of the rush of blood. By closing the upper area, the vessels signal that they have had enough and that other body parts should have their turn. The pressure on the lower areas increases in turn as the upper portions shut down. This is what happens with all the related consequences when the psyche preferentially concentrates on the upper masculine area; the conscious mind must release this preference and then be able to open up to the opposite pole as well.

In this respect, it is not at all surprising that men feel the effects of the coarctation of the aorta three times more frequently than women. They naturally tend to emphasize their masculinity superficially without confronting it in its more meaningful depths, and they are naturally more afraid of the consuming depths of the feminine. As long as they can remain aware of this, it will be emotionally difficult for them. However, they bring physically dangerous repercussions upon themselves when they do not deal with it consciously.

5.3 Constrictions and Leaking Spots

The term *heart defect* clearly shows that this is an imperfection within one's own center—that something is wrong with the heart. While congenital heart defects can be very diverse, the acquired symptoms concentrate, above all, on two basic themes: the constriction (stenosis) of the heart valves and a state of leakiness (insufficiencies). Since the heart is the center of the circle (the circulatory system) both types of defects have

The Defective Heart

a long-term effect on the entire system and impact both the forward and backward directions of the circular blood flow.

5.3.1 Stenoses or Bottlenecks

When stenosis occurs, the part of the heart that is ahead of the constriction must counteract the obstruction. It therefore becomes stronger in order to master the additional work. If it is not successful in pressing the arriving volume of blood through the congested areas, a backup is inevitable, creating substantial problems for these areas of the circulatory system. In contrast, the areas beyond the constriction are often relieved to the point that they recede as if they were untrained muscles. That is, they lose their strength. The image of the blood flowing through such a constriction can be compared to river rapids or water churning through a narrow gorge. The pressure increases, the current becomes more torrential, and eddies and whirlpools form with all the intrinsic, catastrophic dangers.

Once again, the symbolism of the constriction will point in the direction of fear. Even the allusion to a gorge with its narrow walls and the thundering of its constrained tumult of water can create anxiety. The compressed quantities of blood induce a very similar sound—called *crescendo murmurs*—when they race through the rapids of the vessels. The river (blood) fights against the resistance that the narrowed canyons (vessel walls) offer. The patient affected by a constriction in the heart must admit to himself that there is considerable resistance within his heart; his vitality (symbolized by the blood) is up in arms against this restriction. The *river of life* is obstructed at this central point. If the person in question does not succeed in creating a balance with this obstruction, vitality will become congested and block other areas of life. The basic problem is a lack of openness for the flow of life.

Mitral stenosis; The mitral stenosis between the left heart atrium and the left ventricle strains the atrium. This may lead to an expansion, with the associated danger of atrium fibrillation due to hypertrophy—for example, excessive tissue and organ enlargement. Within normal limits, such narrowing is compensated through an extended influx of blood. However, when the heart receives additional stress causing an increase in the pulse rate or heartbeat, this compensation is no longer possible. As a result, the patient can hardly withstand strain because his center can no longer deal with the increased demands. In this case, the lungs are affected by the backed up fluid and this can lead to the secretion of congested fluids into the air passages, perhaps resulting in pulmonary edema. If the congestion is chronic, a constriction of the pulmonary vessels can occur because of the increased pressure in the pulmonary circulatory system. The result of this is a strain on the right heart, which must now pump against the resistance in the lungs.

Even before the development of such a regurgitation of the right heart, the patient suffers from severe disabilities. Because of the reduced flow of blood, his body continually suffers from too little energy and the blood supplies very little oxygen to the cells; hence, the patient has a tendency to turn blue (cyanosis). People affected by this symptom are generally pale. In the case of strain, dizziness and fainting can occur because the energy supply is inadequate. In addition, exertion quickly leads to a shortness of breath. The resulting symptoms of so-called congestive bronchitis intensify and these symptoms sometimes even include coughing up blood. A desperate attempt by the body for compensation can be seen by an increased production of red blood corpuscles (polycythemia). Even if the body is no longer able to keep the stream of life flowing adequately, it will make the blood as nutritious as possible.

From this impressive clinical picture, the psychological theme is revealed. The afflicted one must have been so frightened at one time that she did not want to admit this to herself and now this lack of insight is making a troublesome course throughout the body. An obstruction in the center of her own life is suffocating her, and this hindrance in her own center devours a great deal of vitality and leaves the patient without any reserves. She can no longer afford any type of physical exertion without having justifiable fear for her survival. Under these conditions, the body reflects how pale life has become, as hot red (the color of vitality) has turned to cool blue (the color that has always indicated a lack of energy and lifelessness). If the patient does not honestly admit to her frailties but acts as though she is still a match for the demands of life, her heart will very quickly expose the swindle and she will become dizzy and—if necessary—she will faint to indicate her true distress. The shortness of breath that also occurs at such times demonstrates that the central obstacle in life extends beyond the heart to the level of communication. Together with the heart, the lungs are our most important organ of communication and exchange. In addition to the gaseous transaction, they also guarantee our spoken communication. However, this exchange is obstructed. Instead of words that flow from the heart, the afflicted person coughs up blood. This, naturally, also comes from the heart—a congested heart. In addition, the coughing illustrates an aggressive component—the patient is spewing out her heart's blood at the surrounding world.

In the case of the angina-pectoris patient, everything revolves around the narrowness of the heart and the fear which lies behind this condition. In this case, bottlenecks involve the supply of blood to the heart which illustrates that the heart is not being fed enough in the figurative sense. In mitral stenosis, the bottleneck does not only affect the supply of blood to the heart—it affects the supply to the entire body. The victim must admit that his vital energy cannot flow freely and that the body has paid for it with a chronic energy crisis that becomes more threatening with every challenge. The body already forces the patient into decisive insights. He must learn to accept his limitations. The stenosis limits the vital flow, thereby restricting him. The symptom demands renunciation and recognition of these limits and every slight effort reminds the patient of them.

Projecting these images on the emotional level is the patient's primary task. Only when he recognizes his own narrow emotional limitations—and the barriers that obstruct his life in the figurative sense—will he have the chance for relief on the physical level. By accepting his emotional helplessness (which the physical fainting spells reflect) and by seeing through his swindle (in every demonstration of power) the proper attitude corresponding to the limited situation in life can develop. An aggressive stance is out of the question. There is no room for compensating with a cocky attitude; faintheartedness is nothing more than the unresolved aspect of the task. The crux of the matter is ultimately learning to be humble. Even in pictorial terms, life forces the victim to his knees—to a posture that connotes humility and submission more than anything else.

Only if one masters these primary learning tasks can the strength develop to integrate the opposite attitude into life—bringing with it an expansiveness and a free flow of energy. Initially, this must take place on the emotional level and is even easier to translate into action. If this step is lacking and the problem is only approached on the physical level by exploding the bottleneck in a surgical procedure, complications will be more than likely. The left ventricle has felt too little strain for a long time; it may no longer be capable of dealing with the unaccustomed burden of normal blood flow. Another possible complication is the *postcommissurotomy syndrome* (the body's quasi-allergic reaction to the operation).

However, the clear symptoms and the subsequent serious operation frequently have their own impressive psychotherapeutic effect. The entire theme of undergoing an operation demands that the patient admit helplessness after having recognized the fact that she can no longer help herself. She consciously surrenders to the helpless state under anesthesia, showing clearly that her own consciousness is only a disruptive factor to her health and, therefore, must be switched off completely. Even the act of subjecting oneself to the knife requires a rather strong awareness of the situation. When the consciousness has experienced all of these steps, the surgeon may reopen the proper passageway to renew the stream of life. Naturally, this applies in essence to all surgeries; they always indicate the patient's

The Defective Heart

capitulation of his own forces; surgery is also held in reserve for distinct emergencies only.

Mitral stenosis occurs four times more frequently in women than in men. From this statistic one may conclude that women have a much more difficult time allowing their vital energies to flow freely, or women may run into obstacles in this process more frequently than men. On the other hand, it might also be that it is more difficult for women to admit such obstacles to themselves on a conscious level and they may tend to push these problems aside.

Aortic stenosis: The aortic valve between the left heart and the main artery can become a bottleneck. In at least half of the cases, this heart defect is congenital. For the other half, the cause is rheumatic endocarditis. A geriatric form may also be diagnosed, but this is due to sclerosis (hardening) in the valve. The noises at these rapids are even more impressive. In addition to a loud, raw explosive sound, the heartbeat has increased. Instead of the normal two beats, as many as four may occur in the same time. The pressure in the left heart increases enormously, but it drops off dramatically at the valve barrier so that the blood pressure and pulse are weak. For ninety percent of the patients, the narrow spot calcifies with time.

The extent of the heart's compensatory abilities is indicated by the fact that the symptoms first occur when the valve opening has shrunk to one quarter of its original size. Even then, the compensatory possibilities of the heart are not at all exhausted. The left heart can increase in strength to such a degree that it may continue to function for more than thirty or forty years practically without manifesting any symptoms. However, when it does strike up against the limitations of the extended stress, the patient usually has very few years left to live.

If the left heart no longer succeeds in performing its work, a regurgitation with ventricle enlargement and congestion in the lungs develops. In this case, the signs correspond to those of mitral stenosis, ranging from pale skin to shortness of breath; the danger of pulmonary edema—and ultimately the failure of the right heart—is imminent. As a special characteristic, aortic stenosis strain can also trigger angina-pectoris attacks that may intensify into a heart attack—in addition to all of the familiar signs. On the physical level, the reason for this is the anatomy of the heart. The coronary arteries start at the very beginning of the aorta; they thereby become caught up in an alarming dilemma. On the one hand, due to the enlargement of the left heart ventricle, they have taken on additional supply work; on the other hand, they receive blood with very little pressure, because of the enormous loss of pressure at the bottleneck and their location just after the barrier. The extended time for expulsion and the increased pressure in the left ventricle additionally obstruct their work. If there is even more strain, an increase in the amount of energy is required; this creates pain at the threshold in the truest sense of the word.

For aortic stenosis, the problems addressed under mitral stenosis and angina pectoris consequently merge. Neither the body nor the heart receive enough nutrition. The unconscious emotional theme in the background thereby signals that the emotional level of the heart—as well as the flow of vital energy—is threatening to become exhausted. One may imagine the metaphor of a central water pump that supplies a large garden through a system of irrigation ditches. In the case of aortic stenosis, a bottleneck exists at the beginning of the main canal that routes the freshly pumped water outward. However, because of this bottleneck, the pump itself is also deprived of water so that its output becomes increasingly weak. This image illustrates the interlinking of the various processes and how the problems build upon one another. Because of the bottleneck, the pump has to produce a greater output. However, the bottleneck itself reduces its ability to work properly. Although its water supply requirements are higher under this additional strain, it is precisely the strain itself that reduces the water supply. Such a situation necessarily leads to catastrophe.

The image on the emotional level functions according to very similar criteria. One unresolved problem usually results in further problems. If one looks at the various areas of the irrigation system, one observes that each of them has more than enough reasons for failure. These reasons can always be located outside each area of responsibility. For example, the pump could easily demand from the supply pipes that they provide at least an adequate supply, since the pump has to work harder. With the same degree of justification, the pipes could stipulate that they cannot function under such additional demand if the blood comes to them under higher pressure.

Even though this may be quite easy to comprehend on a symbolic level, the person in question faces a bigger difficulty to achieve this understanding. The person even sets conditions before he begins dealing with those problems. However, in both—the examples of an irrigation system and of aortic stenosis—one can easily recognize that this is not the right time to set conditions. They do not end the conflict but instead lead more deeply into a vicious cycle. It is usually quite inappropriate to react with mandated conditions or demands to a problem that has already reached the body level. On the basis of the inner logic of the entire process, such behavior can only lead deeper into the entanglement. This can become particularly clear for complex problems like aortic stenosis. All heart defects are ultimately very well suited for seeing through this complexity because, through the circulatory system, they also affect other organs such as the lungs and liver.

Within this context, it may become obvious that even any form of advantage through the illness—such as the necessarily reduced stress for heart patients—is extremely detrimental. In addition to dedication and responsibility for oneself, the step towards healing always requires relinquishing all emotional leniency that a person has created for himself by not working through the learning tasks at hand.

The therapy for aortic stenosis prescribed by orthodox medicine consists of the operative exploding of the bottleneck or the replacement of the valve with a prosthesis. That such a replacement alone cannot offer the necessary relief is shown in the required subsequent treatment. Although the prosthesis keeps the aorta open, the danger of the formation of thrombosis and of an even more severe embolism is a result. For this reason, after such an operation, patients must use agents for blood liquefaction (anticoagulants) for the rest of their lives.[15]

The stream of vital energy shows these problems in yet another manner. With the violence of surgery, the barrier has been removed from the physical setting; the director now has to think of a new stage so that the impending theme will come into the limelight. The formation of thrombosis, blood clots, and swirls on the artificial valve will fulfill this purpose precisely. The blood clots are carried into the body through the blood stream and may lead to an embolism by clogging vessels somewhere else in the body. The theme of obstructing the stream of life thereby continues to exist. The liquefaction of the blood attempts to achieve what in the long term must occur on the emotional level: keeping the vital stream flowing and preventing stoppages and blocks.

In this sense, the patient receives a further prosthesis that physically takes over the job that he has not prepared for or is not capable of performing on the emotional level. The *prosthesis* placed in the foreground will obstruct the patient's view of his actual task. Considered from another perspective, the patient hides behind the prosthesis; he probably hopes that no one will notice that he is missing something essential.

A further effect of the artificial valve contributes to greater honesty; this is the hemalysis that occurs. This is a literal dissolution of the blood or the destruction of the red blood cells at the prosthesis. However, the red blood cells transport the oxygen—connected to the iron molecules—and therefore symbolize the vital energy to a special degree. Their dissolution and corresponding loss of iron illustrates how much this involves the issue of vitality. The extent of the hemalysis reaction differs greatly in each patient since the surgeon cannot predict how the hemalysis will manifest itself and this demonstrates how much leeway still remains for the *director* or the *inner* physician to implement the necessary themes.

Tricuspidal stenosis: The stenosis of the tricuspidal valve, between the right atrium and the right ventricle, occurs less frequently and appears, above all, in combination with a mitral stenosis. Like the latter, it is usually the result of a rheumatic fever, which is seldom congenital, and it occurs in women more frequently than in men. The result is inadequate circulation in the lungs with cyanosis (turning blue) during exertion; however, it is primarily a considerable backing up of blood into the venous system. Because of the greater receptivity of the veins, the pressure on the heart is much less than in the case of mitral stenosis. The main symptoms are found in the organs affected by the buildup—most of all in the liver. It can be so congested that the palpating hand can actually feel pulsations within it. Although the effects on the heart itself are not very impressive, life expectancy is very limited if one does not take the necessary measures both emotionally and physically.

In this case, the heart is not open for the returning blood. Expressed another way, one's own center does not adequately open up to the vital stream and partially rejects it. This problem is not consciously confronted; therefore, the emotional theme sinks into the body where it repeatedly offers itself as a symptom to be treated. The congestion of one's vital energy becomes particularly conspicuous in the liver—the organ that symbolically represents the reconnecting of the human being with his very source (the *religio*)—and, thereby, the patient is at issue with the meaning of life. The inference about this symbolic significance results from the function of the liver. It disassembles the ingested plant and animal protein down to the amino acids (the basic building blocks of life) and reconstructs protein specific to human beings from it. The individual amino acids are the same in plants, animals, and humans—as is the genetic code with which they correlate to their respective typical proteins. Consequently, there is a common level to all life and so we all share a connection at the deepest source—the origin. With this buildup in the liver, the vital energy points to the themes of religion and philosophy—philosophy in its original meaning as the love of wisdom. This is the theme of congested veins with the vanishing of *the vital nectar,* which is urgently needed somewhere else. This was outlined in detail in Section II.II on the circulatory system

The learning task for the patient consists of becoming aware of the theme "lack of openness for the vital stream," admitting to oneself that one has shut oneself off from the stream of life or narrowed oneself to its tides.

Even the heart defect alone shows that it is not possible to demand the opposite pole immediately—namely the openness of oneself First, it is a matter of accepting and resolving the principle portrayed by the symptom which, in this case, is frugality in dealing with the life energies and a wise restriction to the essential. The restricted circulation in the lungs suggests that too little energy flows into the area of communication. This means becoming aware of the inadequate treatment of a central theme. Instead of forcing oneself to do the opposite in the form of cramped conversation, there is also the possibility of seeking quietness and solitude. However, the congestion also shows where something has to happen—where the attention should accumulate or be concentrated. It would, therefore, be appropriate to concern oneself with the purpose of one's own life and with life in general, instead of longing for or even demanding the expanse and abundance of the opposite pole. This can be done ideally during those times of forced conscious silence.

Pulmonary stenosis: Pulmonary stenosis narrows the exit from the right heart into the lungs and leads to similar manifestations such as the constriction of the tricuspidal valve that resides merely one station ahead of it in the blood stream. However, in this case the cardiac strain lies more in the foreground since the obstacle is not at the entrance to the heart but at its exit. This means that the heart itself lies within the congestive area, causing the heart with its associated themes to shift more strongly into the focus of attention. Instead of *congesting* within the physical heart, the vital energy should be *concentrated* on the typical themes of the heart.

5 3.2 Regurgitations or Leaking Valves

A leaking valve is the opposite pole to valves with constrictions or stenoses. Yet, both types of defects lead (as is so often the case with opposite poles) to very similar results—increased work for the heart. Too little or too much openness in the heart creates the same misery: more work with little effect. When the closing of the valve no longer functions, the heart has to perform a true Sisyphean task. It has the same problem as the pitiable hero of Greek mythology who, as a punishment, had to roll a heavy rock up a mountain. However, as soon as he came close to the top, he could no longer hold the stone, and it rolled back down the mountain he had just climbed with such great difficulty. Without allowing himself to take a break, Sisyphus had to continue with his frustrating work. The same thing happens to the heart with leaking valves. By using all of its strength, the heart has barely pushed out the blood stream almost completely, when the blood turns around again and flows back into chamber it just came from, forced out of with so much effort. Despite the frustrating effect of its work, the heart cannot permit itself to take a pause. Instead, it must function without stopping and continue to pump with an even greater effort. Fortunately, not the entire blood stream flows back in, otherwise the victim would die immediately, because no progress is possible within the circulatory system any longer.

With the next contraction of the heart muscle, the blood that has flowed back in must also be managed. This results in a stretching of the affected heart areas. However, every expansion increases the strength of the heart through a reflex mechanism so that the organ—independent of the returning stream's proportions—must perform a considerable amount of additional work. Practically speaking, the returning blood must be pumped several times. In this sense, one may compare such a heart with a mountaineer who climbs a steep slope in deep snow. After two steps forwards, he always slips one step backwards. He is lacking in support for every step, just as the defective heart does not have the necessary backing for each of its actions. If one has ever climbed a mountain in the snow, one will know how much increased effort and torment occurs with such inhibited progress.

On the figurative level, it is justifiable to suspect a non-conscious problem. The patient unconsciously is in the same situation as the mountain climber who is totally concerned with the "progress" of his ascent but suffers because of the many little steps backwards. Every time his life stream flows in a forward direction, he pays for it with substantial steps backwards. Because he does not want to perceive these backwards steps (also called regressions in the emotional area), they must manifest on the physical stage. The patient is lacking the necessary support in life. He is open in all directions, including those that do not help him advance but hold him back. Even where it would be urgently necessary, he cannot close himself off. The result is that things that should remain separated cannot remain isolated from each other any longer. Because of the exaggerated openness, the power of differentiation suffers, primarily concerning one's own vital energy. It is not the openness itself that is misguided, but it appears at the wrong moment and in the wrong direction. The direction is practically reversed. A person moves backward instead of forward and does not even realize the fact—only because the heart is groaning as a result of the additional strain.

Openness may be a lofty objective, but an undifferentiated openness in a polarized world is only possible in a state of illumination, if at all. In the general physical realm and the normal emotional realm, an appropriate amount of reserve is required. Just as the valves in the heart must hold in order to give the blood stream the necessary support for its progress, in the figurative sense it is important for a person to "shut one's trap" once in a while and say no, holding back at the right moment. Folk wisdom is aware of this problem when it tells us: the most difficult thing in life is to say no! Only if it is possible to do so, can one be successful in providing one's own vital energy with the necessary support. In contrast, a person who can never hold back and is unable to say no must perform a great deal of senseless work, just as the heart does. Such openness will certainly be taken advantage of and, as a result, the person will often work/or *nothing* in both senses of the word. Instead of making progress on the path in life, one must encounter setbacks. The blood and the heart may just be more honest, but they struggle with exactly the same problem. Therefore, every heartbeat also brings a major or minor setback and, instead of flowing forward, the life stream seems to run on the spot. Despite vehement activity, the blood and the patient do not budge from the spot or in any case do not get very far, neither within the circulatory system nor in life. Perceiving this tendency within life's central matters is the best opportunity for providing relief to the heart and circulation.

Heart valves that are leaking naturally may also indicate that the afflicted person is not clear within himself, on the figurative level. That is also closely associated with the lack of ability to say no. When an individual cannot set boundaries and is not able to hold back, he will quickly let himself be pulled in the wrong direction as well. This is illustrated precisely by inadequate support causing the misdirection of the blood.

After such an admission, which is certainly not easy to make, the next step should be dedicated to the voluntary resolution of the theme. This may be accomplished through a conscious retraction of the vital energy—paying attention to what one might receive as compared with what one has expended. The symptom itself already forces a slower progress on the physical level. Also, taking it to heart in the figurative sense can only develop from the acceptance of the corresponding learning tasks. A slower progress, that requires being more conscious of the required efforts, automatically brings more deliberation into play and, therefore, establishes the initial basis for the ability to differentiate later.

However, the central theme remains the openness that one must preserve and consciously guide into the right direction. It is first necessary to be open to one's own steps backwards. Regressions in the emotional area are steps backwards on stages of development that a person has already left behind but prefers to repeat again, out of fear* of the new steps that are now at hand. Such clinging to themes that have long been outdated are comparable to the alcoholic reaching for the bottle in all difficult situations. This reflexive reaching out is completely correct for the infant, but for an adult it is a step backwards that prevents further progress. A conscious openness for such shrinking back from the new path, the new task, offers the opportunity to discover this safe but no longer appropriate level as a stepping stone on the path into new territory. We can only really progress from the point where we are.

Ultimately, this can also mean to go back consciously in one's own life and on a higher level, to follow one's own tracks so to speak. Similar to the Prodigal Son from the Bible who must turn around and return home once he has perceived his failure, and similar to Parsival who had to experience his own life backward in time in order to become truly mature for the decisive question: "Uncle, what is your problem?" This question is naturally advisable for all symptoms. In the case of heart defects, and especially the regurgitations with their retreat problems, it is particularly important.

Only if reconciliation with the principle portrayed in the clinical picture is successful, the opposite pole, which means free progress, and the necessary support for this step can be realized. The legend of the Holy Grail illustrates that everything comes in its own time. In his youth and long before the theme of return is relevant at all, Parsival makes use of the reserve learned at home from his mother Herzeloide and asks no questions during his first visit to the Castle of the Holy Grail, causing him to miss his task completely. It was much too early for such polite reserve, because his task still was to conquer the world. In this same manner, the patient must first learn correct openness and permeability at the right moment, through the valvular regurgitation of his heart, before he can mature to use the reserve that is necessary as well.

Mitral regurgitation: Frequently, mitral regurgitation is connected with a stenosis; different combinations of heart defects manifest quite often. However, in this case the problem multiplies itself. The entire matter can be easily understood on the physical level. As a result of rheumatic fever, a shrinking and scarring of the valve and the tendinous fibers that hold it can naturally lead to constriction and leaks at the same time. On the emotional level, the interpretations for the two problems are combined. The problems are more serious and easily get out of hand, as the corresponding symptoms reveal in the following.

When a failure of the mitral valve occurs, during the heart contraction a portion of the blood flows out of the left ventricle back into the left atrium and threatens to congest back into the lungs. However, for a long period of time this heart defect can be compensated by the left ventricle's large reserve capacity. When the left heart starts to develop signs of weakness, there is a quick occurrence of pulmonary congestion and subsequent failure of the right heart that progresses much more rapidly than on the opposite side. This fundamentally life-threatening situation is also illustrated by the very high risk of an attempted operation. On the other hand, if an operation is postponed for too long, its prospects are even worse. The significance of this fact has already been outlined in the above. In addition, complications with the lungs, as the communication organ, may occur and have to be taken into consideration.

Aortic regurgitation: For two out of three patients, aortic regurgitation can be traced back to rheumatic fever. This number is three times higher for men than for women. Only mitral valve regurgitation can be compensated better by the heart, due to the enormous reserve powers of the left ventricle. However, these reserves are now considerably in demand. The amount of blood that flows back into the left ventricle from the aorta may even be as high as the normal volume of a healthy heart. In this case, a substantial enlargement of the heart is necessary in order to deal with the oversized flooding of blood. The medical profession calls this *cor bovinum* (ox heart). The elastic receptive powers of the aorta, that give the blood stream its continuity in the normal case and largely compensate for the pressure difference between the contraction and relaxation phases, fail completely because of the defect. Because of the valvular defect, the considerably enlarged pressure difference is transferred without correction to the entire circulatory system. Even when he is at rest, the patient feels his heart beating, his face is flushed, the carotid artery pulsates and reveals the high level of tension. Since the pulse rate is very strong and fast, the blood in the capillaries of the finger tips and in the carotids pulsate, the head nods in the rhythm of the pulse which one can virtually see. Doctors call this condition a *homo pulsans,* a pulsating human being. Through the enormous loss of pressure during the heart's relaxation phase, angina-pectoris attacks can occur in addition since the coronary vessels no longer receive an adequate supply of blood. However, it is precisely these vessels which are dependent on an adequate blood supply in the relaxation phase. Since the blood pressure in this phase practically suffers a total collapse, this results also in a lack of pressure in these pipelines.

The picture of the pulsating person dramatically illustrates the interpretations that are theoretically derived in the above. The constant nodding of the head to the rhythm of the heart symbolizes the basic emotional attitude of constant openness in all directions and the notorious yes-man stance. Wherever this person turns, he already nods in advance without even being asked. One can even observe the immense amount of work performed completely in vain of his center. He pulsates and vibrates with activity, but nothing leads to a result. Not only does the marking of time become obvious in his constantly flushed face, but also in the running in place that does not bring him forward one bit despite all his efforts. This basic attitude (described in the sections on angina pectoris and the heart attack) aptly completes this picture, as well as the fact that men are affected three times more frequently than women.

This last statistical indication may throw additional light on the diligence and correctness of the magnificent director's work

The Defective Heart

behind the scenes. In most of the cases, both mitral stenosis and aortic regurgitation can be traced back to the same basic conflict. This conflict is concretely represented by rheumatic fever. Considered from the perspective of the physical stage, almost the same props (antigens) are used in order to perform pieces dealing with problems that are virtually the opposite of each other but still revolve around the same basic theme of openness. The difference in the distribution of gender very well reflects the social circumstances, and, therefore, this distribution could not appear differently in this society.

Tricuspidal regurgitation: The valvular defect between the right atrium and the right ventricle leads to an increased strain on the right heart, which reacts with much more sensitivity to this problem than the left heart. Through the constant flow back into the right atrium and from there into the venous system, an increase in pressure occurs, even with a downright venous pulse. While, in the case of aortic regurgitation, the carotid arteries pulsate, now the jugular veins pulsate. The only sensible direction of flow is obviously reversed. Where one normally encounters tranquil repose and a peacefully flowing blood stream on its way to the heart, now there are disturbances lashing out. The expression "to be full of hot air" comes up, a person who creates hot air, resulting in disturbances in the flow in places where it does not belong. In fact, the result only signifies a questionable sign of activity. A person like this engages in useless activities with no obvious purpose or with "much ado about nothing."

The backup into the venous system leads, as already mentioned in the section on tricuspidal stenosis, to congestion of the liver in those pulsations that one can feel. In the long term, it results in the so-called cardiac liver, a life-threatening chronic transformation process of the liver. Once again, the themes of *religio* and life philosophy are addressed through the liver.

Furthermore, the backup leads to edemas in the lower parts of the body and the formation of ascites, that is the leakage of tissue fluid into body cavities. It is then possible that a small lake will form in the abdominal cavity. When the physician taps the abdomen, a real wave phenomenon can be triggered and the formation of ascites can be found. Symbolically, water is the classical element of the soul and the emotions. It is the most feminine among the four elements. Water that is backing up signifies that the patient can no longer integrate the feminine-emotional qualities into the flow of life. They are pressed against and through the (vessel) walls and thereby relegated to the available sidetracks. It is understandable that an individual cannot exist for long without these qualities. On the physical level, the patient is already missing the protein bound in the tissue fluid, protein that is the fundamental building substance of the human body.

Pulmonary regurgitation: Pulmonary regurgitation practically never occurs by itself. Instead, it appears as relative regurgitation accompanying a severe mitral stenosis or so-called pulmonary hypertension, high blood pressure in the pulmonary circulation.

6.

The Heart Out of Rhythm

The fact that the heartbeat determines life's rhythms can be observed when it breaks out of its usual harmony. When the heart races, a flood of emotions and impressions overwhelm the patient and life accelerates its tempo. If a person's heart stumbles, she immediately feels herself thrown out of rhythm. Apart from such moments, the heart rhythm is so familiar and so completely adapted to the respective needs of the body and soul that one hardly notices. This self-evident and unconscious feeling for the heart is further increased by the autonomy of its beat that eludes willful influence to a very large extent. A certain degree of control over the heart can be achieved only through intensive autogenous training or biofeedback. Even then, it remains considerably more difficult to influence the heart beat than, for example, the breathing rhythm, which one can willfully force out of its autonomy at any time. The rhythm of the heart is consequently an expression of a strict and independent norm of the body.

However, beyond those acute situations the heart determines the life rhythm in a much deeper sense. Children's hearts beat more quickly than those of older people, and, therefore, the life rhythm of children is enhanced as well. Parallel to this situation, the children experience the flow of time in a distinctly slower manner—or, expressed in a different way: the first ten years of childhood pass slowly, the next ten years of adolescence go by somewhat quicker and so on up into the later decades of life that practically seem to fly by. The quicker the heart beats, the more intensely time is experienced. This makes the heart the human being's inner clock, measuring his lifetime.

The heart not only strikes the individual hour for human beings, it also has this same task in the animal kingdom. According to objective time measurement, a fly only lives for three weeks. However through the incomparably high frequency of its life rhythm, this short time is stretched out enormously in subjective terms. The fly's unbelievably fast reaction time alone proves how much it can achieve during this "short" time. From its perspective, humans live in a slow-motion world, that is why catching flies can be such a strenuous task. The larger the life forms are, the slower their life rhythm is. The heart of the placid elephant only beats twenty-five times a minute, but the animal reaches an age of more than sixty years.

The correlation between the heart frequency and the flow of time may become even clearer through an example from modem medical research. Many patients who have experienced a life-threatening accident report that, seconds before, the occurrence stretched out into a true eternity, and that many things went through their minds. Sometimes, they saw their entire lives pass by as if it were a film. What subjectively appeared to take a long time happened objectively and within fractions of a second. On the physical level during these moments, the body is inundated with adrenaline, the stress hormone that puts the sympathetic nervous system into a state of high tension and forces the heart to race. In such objectively short and yet subjectively long periods of time, the ability to react is enormously increased. This may also lead to such things as admirable rescue measures. A similar situation is probably experienced by predatory animals, that have a considerably higher level of adrenaline than herbivores, while they hunt.

The Heart Out of Rhythm

If one's heart stands completely still, the flow of one's lifetime changes not only quantitatively but also qualitatively. In the moment of the cardiac standstill, the lifetime objectively ends, but subjectively an entirely new time begins with experiences that one can hardly comprehend from the perspective of linear time flow. People who have been pulled back from the threshold of death by means of modem intensive-care medicine report an experience somewhat similar to that of a film that lets their lives pass in review before their inner eye. Deeply religious experiences, as described in the holy books of various cultures, are also possible within this time span. Books of the dead, such as those of Tibet and the Egypt, present impressive accounts of the world beyond the heart rhythm.

The secret of the heartbeat lies in a highly ingenious combination of normal heart muscle cells and those which have specialized in conducting stimulation. In pictorial terms, the heart can be compared to a completely interconnected country of the future. In this picture, the sinus node in the atrium area would be the broadcasting center, setting the tone for the entire country. It has a resting frequency of sixty to eighty beats per minute. However, this signal is not transmitted directly to all households or cells, but further distributed through a sophisticated system. Only the muscle cells of the atria receive the signal directly since they must start with their work first. The corresponding rhythm is transmitted further through three central and considerably quicker pathways to a subsequent second transmission station, the atrioventricular node, which it reaches even before the signal arrives at the individual cells of the atrium. There, the information is held back until the atria can finish their work ahead of the ventricles. From the atrioventricular node, the impulse runs through the fast-conducting fibers to the tip of the heart, while it simultaneously goes through the slow conduction paths directly from the atrioventricular nodes to the surrounding cells. This guarantees the stimulation of all ventricle cells at the right moment and so they can begin their mutual work synchronously.

Ultimately, each muscle cell is connected to the broadcasting center. However, this takes place within a carefully coordinated hierarchy that ensures that all participants will receive the information at the proper time. The strict adherence to this hierarchy is an indispensable prerequisite for the heart to function flawlessly. In the process, the origin of the word hierarchy quite clearly reveals what this means for the heart. Composed of the two Greek words, *hieros,* meaning filled with divine power, holy, and *árchein,* meaning to be the first, or to rule, the word hierarchy represents the dominion of the holy or the idea that what is holy belongs at the beginning. In the heart, the divine or initial power is symbolized by the sinus node, which rules unchallenged in normal situations. It is the natural pacemaker and so strong that when it acts, it deprives all other cells of their power. This is necessary because the sinus node is the first among its equals and must not neglect its leadership role for a single moment. If it fails even once to deprive the others of their power in time, it will immediately create competition. A cell that is lower in the hierarchy will take over command until the sinus node reclaims its position with a new demonstration of power. Number two in the hierarchy is the atrioventricular node that manages forty to fifty beats a minute, and number three are the so-called Purkinje's fibers that conduct the impulse from the atrioventricular node into the tip of the heart. They can attain a pulse rate of twenty to forty beats a minute, which is barely adequate for life. If this impulse-giver were to fail as well, the common heart cells could create a pulse on their own, but this would not achieve much because their rate is too low.

One may say that the subordinate centers in the hierarchy are always waiting their turn. After every action of the heart, they once again prepare for deployment. Only the stronger action of the sinus node forces them time and again to calm down and merely serve as information bearers. In the image of the interconnected country, this means that the various subordinate broadcasting stations, whose purpose is to convey the information, constantly prepare programs of their own. These must be cancelled by the central broadcasting station at any instant. Within the sound heart, this action creates positive competition that, in a normal situation, has no negative effect because of a healthy hierarchy. However as soon as the dominion of the *"holy" (the center) demonstrates weakness, a revolution breaks out, and the next highest degree of rank in the pyramid demands its rights. It is then that the medical profession speaks of a substitutive rhythm.

The regulation of the heart is supported in essence by the sinus node, but the sinus node itself, as well as its rhythm, is very strongly dependent on emotional and physical influences. As soon as one meets an emotional or physical challenge, the heart rate increases and conversely, when one calms down again eventually, the heart rate slows down accordingly. The parallelism of the emotional and the physical state is especially clear when one considers the heart. If, for example, a person feels aggressive, it is not unusual for the heart "to be in the mouth." If one then does attack, the additional energy made available by to the increased work of the heart is beneficial. If a person immerses himself in a state of spiritual-emotional repose, such as meditation, the heart rate is measurably reduced, and the body needs less energy.

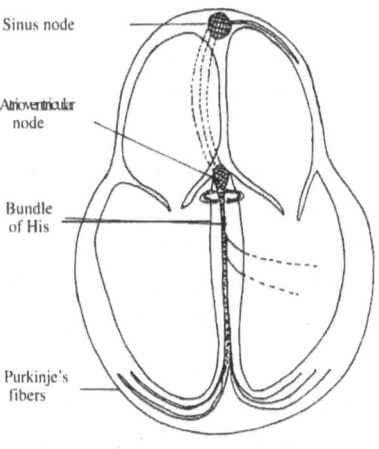

Illustration 4

On the physiological level, these effects are imparted through the two poles of the autonomous nervous system and its corresponding hormones. The nerves of the sympathetic nervous system and the catecholamines[16] increase the excitability of the sinus node by facilitating its discharge or depolarization. On the other hand, nerves of the opposite pole, the vagus nerves, reduce the excitability of the node by impeding electrical depolarization under the influence of the hormone acetylcholine. Therefore, agitation increases the heart rate as well as the blood pressure, while deep states of relaxation reduce both the blood pressure and the heart rate.

Palpitations (bradyarrhythmia) are a part of our everyday life and everybody experiences them to a certain degree. Every emotion influences the heart rate, and every intense emotion contorts the moderate rhythm of the heart. It may be a fright that lets the heart stand still (in the figurative sense) and causes it to skip a beat, perhaps it is panic that causes it to race, or joy that lets it beat faster. The heart and emotions form an inseparable unity, and each emotion is reflected in the heart. In the same way that a Geiger counter reacts to radioactivity, the heart reacts to emotions and registers them with sensitive precision. A seismograph, that records the tremors within the earth, from the weakest shift to volcanic eruptions and earthquakes, is an even better metaphor. The heart also registers everything from the smallest emotional impulse to emotional outbursts and heartbreaks.

Within certain limits, the heart should certainly leap out of its accustomed harmony. It should jump for joy within the body, and even a certain anxiety around the heart is in order if the corresponding emotional situation is an oppressive experience. Those situations which are medical cardiac arrhythmia deal with a very similar occurrence, but the patient no longer experiences the emotions. He does not admit them to himself or to his conscious mind, and therefore they sink into the body and there obtain the attention they need. Consequently, people who are frequently aware of their emotions and feelings and who are open to irrational emotional eruptions in their daily lives, do not need to reckon with palpitations. However, those who depend completely upon their rational minds and are not themselves bothered by emotions, may easily disrupt their routine by the cardiac arrhythmia.

When an individual's heart acts up, he should ask himself if he only rarely permits himself to "act up" in life. His life has possibly been squeezed into rigid tracks. Static principles have imposed their even tempo on his life. Insurance has provided security for all uncertainties and there is simply nothing left that could throw this person off the track and nothing that could displace his strict standards. In this case, the heart remains as the final shriek that puts an end to false certainties. When an individual secures life against any type of emotional assault, because he closes his heart to such impulses, he at the same time unconsciously opens his physical heart for the corresponding attacks. Therefore, the afflicted person is then forced to listen once again to his heart and even to obey it for a long lime.

6.1 Problems at the Top of the Hierarchy

Palpitations that originate from the uppermost authority, the sinus node, are very rare. Tachycardia (a racing of the heart) usually accompanies a lack of physical exercise. The untrained heart is disproportionately small and correspondingly weak. When emotional and physical demands increase slightly, it may start to race and, thereby, show how poorly it can cope with any kind of challenge. Raging fears result in the racing of the heart. The heart that is too weak and small unmasks itself as a true hare's heart. The center of the patient is inadequately prepared or simply untrained for life.

Once again, the solution lies in the symptom itself. In the long term, it is a matter of finding the opposite pole or a well-balanced, harmonious rhythm for the heart and the life. However, first it is important to listen to the symptom and obey its requests.

Heart-Aches

A hectic drumming is going on within one's own center, a racing movement. In this case, orthodox therapy clarifies the task at hand and recommends mild exercise in order to accustom the heart gradually to better performance. This is exactly what is involved on the emotional level. Apparently, the racing heart wants to make the person get a move on, wants to bring motion into life and to create inner flexibility. It drives the affected person raving mad, yet it just wants to make him hurry up and come to terms with the feelings in his heart and to allow disorder into his orderly life.

The second therapy proposed by orthodox medicine illustrates this emotional background and consists of the administration of beta blockers. The block of the beta receptors cuts the heart off from all forms of exciting (sympathicotonic) stimulus and thereby prevents the anxious emotions from expressing themselves in the body by means of somatization, which converts emotions into physical symptoms. A similar effect is achieved by tranquilizers, which are the third variation of therapy offered by orthodox medicine. In this case, and in full confidence, the medical field speaks of a psychoautonomous decoupling. The decoupling of soul and intestines, for example, separates the victim from his body and deprives the soul of a further means of expression through the physical body. In the short term, this is completely what the patient wants, since he longs for peace from the emotions that drive him crazy. However in the long term he will slip one step deeper into his dilemma.

As with all symptoms, the galloping heart forces a person to be honest with himself and shows to which liveliness and speed the sufferer has been summoned. The symbolic meaning of the small, weak heart becomes clear when compared to the opposite pole—the large, strong, and therefore, courageous heart.

Heart racing in the case of thyroid hyperactivity has a completely different base. This disturbance does not originate in the heart at all but from the thyroid gland. It signifies a totally whipped-up situation. Not just the heart, but the entire organism, is flooded with hormones that stimulate the metabolism, that

The Heart Out of Rhythm

have the effect of strong stimulants. The patient feels driven, loses weight despite a large appetite, no longer experiences cold, and instead frequently quivers due to physical excitation. Sometimes, the eyes of such an individual also bulge in an odd manner and emphasize the physical hyperactivity. The entire body and its center, the heart, are whipped up. Instead of the racing flight of a hare's heart, this tends more towards the image of the racing reporter whose eyes are almost falling out of his eye sockets due to exaggerated curiosity, and who whips himself up into an extreme state of excitement and perhaps even peps himself up in order to master his daily "very important" work. The heart signals to him the racing frenzy that has seized the center of his life. Such a person really is under the influence of drugs, even if his own body provides them. If we encountered a hunted person in the previous section, we now have a hunter in front of us. That the hare and the hunting dog both have racing hearts is not surprising when one considers the similarities between their physical activity, even if the intentions are exactly the opposite.

The true racing reporter who is aware of his hectic state and who consciously accepts it as a tribute to his profession naturally does not have to suffer from a racing heart. Again, those affected by this condition are only individuals who are not conscious of their racing rhythm in life. In this case, the learning task begins, as usual, with owning up to the extremely turbulent waves within one's own body. Then, there are two possibilities for the next step: the affected individual recognizes that, in the external world, he also stirs up himself and his environment. To the degree that he learns to take responsibility for this, he will also succeed in recognizing the unconscious extremes. Conscious activity will then automatically transform itself from a hectic state into being simply fast, and so the wild chase becomes directed. The unconscious and illness-causing excesses will gradually be resolved. In the second, more difficult case, a piece that is even further away from the patient's consciousness is presented on the wildly animated physical stage of his body. The racing heart and body that is rushing around as if it were a mad thing are the sole evidence for this basic situation, and the outside observer may not have the slightest clue about the drama that's being played out within. As a result, the task of consciously rediscovering the symptoms that have sunk into the body is naturally more difficult, but there is nothing that can replace this task either. Only when the crazy demand has been identified and has been given a chance in life, will the racing of the heart subside.

The image of the racing reporter brings up the idea of work and career, but the theme is not limited to this area. The heart rate can also be affected in a more direct sense, thereby bringing up those emotions associated with love. If a person loses his heart to love, he is either unaware of the extent of the love that he does not yet live, or he does not even admit this love to himself. Because he has forced it out of his consciousness, he no longer even notices it. In both cases, it is naturally a matter of paying attention to the voice of one's own heart and consciously living its message instead of relegating it to the physical heart. With regard to love, there are two "racing" options available. If both of them come together, the result is a virtually classic motif: one person who fears the voice of her heart and flees with a racing heart from somebody else who very well hears his heart's voice but does not realize the entire extent of his love. So he hunts the sweet*heart* who gives his heart no rest and whose heart in the process naturally no longer has any peace either.

6.2 Competition of the Hierarchy

The majority of cardiac arrhythmia are based upon competition in the heart. Some cell of a subordinate center outperforms the sinus node with a higher frequency or a stimulation beginning at an earlier point in time. As long as this form of revolution is successful with the first attempt and another center can establish a new sovereignty, there is no threat to life. However, if instead there is jockeying for the throne and various

The Heart Out of Rhythm

centers attempt to outstrip the others, the work of the heart can be obstructed to the point of heart failure.

The most fortunate situation is always the natural one in which the sinus node sets the tone. In this respect, one can rightly consider the heart to be quite conservative. If another center suddenly plays the first fiddle, this results in problems. However, those problems can remain in check as long as a somewhat workable rhythm arises. The heart can be compared with a rowing eight. Naturally, the ideal situation for the progress of the entire boat is when all eight men unconditionally obey the coxswain. If one member no longer does so and takes over command with a higher number of strokes, it is still better for the others to join him in the new rhythm. However, the new coxswain is certainly not located in the best position to set the stroke. The stem of the boat is the natural location for this purpose since the commander reaches everyone at the same time and from the right direction. If one of the rowers in the middle starts to play the first fiddle, his commands reach the others from different sides and cannot be seen equally well from every point. However, when the new coxswain takes over, the original coxswain is no longer needed. The best thing for him to do is to mind his own business in order not to cause even more confusion.

On the other hand, if none of the rowers is successful in conquering the throne and many of them are seized with the ambition of leadership, the rhythm becomes utter chaos. The opposite of a hierarchy, of the dominion of the holy, occurs; chaos and diversity. Now the individual rowers have greater freedom, and each can continue to row to the best of his ability, but they seem to have forgotten that they are all sitting in the same boat. Perhaps the overall energy that has come into existence is even greater than before, when the mandatory rhythm held back the strongest rowers. Yet, if someone on the shore were to observe the boat, he would see a wild bout of rowing and a total lack of progress. The boat might even sink.

A healthy hierarchy in the heart offers the sole opportunity to achieve wholeness (holiness). If this hierarchy collapses, the

Heart-Aches

affected person must admit to himself that his heart feels torn between conflicting emotions. Irreconcilable endeavors confuse it and block its work. The dominion of the holy, the central meaning of life, has apparently been lost. Without the affected individual having noticed it, a dissipation must have occurred in the essential things at the center of life. Only when the heart begins to beat without any rhythm does it becomes obvious how torn the person is within himself. Then again, the solution cannot be to pull oneself immediately together and concentrate on one thing. It is much more a matter of admitting the conflicting interests and of consciously living them. This is the only way to distinguish the truly central concern among all other interests.

6.3 Paroxysmal Tachycardia— Racing Attacks of the Heart

In addition to the tachycardia that originate at the sinus node, there are also those caused by a competing impulse center. Unlike the type discussed in the previous section, they begin suddenly and drive the heart up to frequencies ranging from 140 to 200 beats per minute. Two basic forms of this affliction can be differentiated by an ECG: a benign form that originates in the atrium, and a variation originating in the ventricle and that indicates an organic defect of the heart muscle.

The abrupt onset of a racing heart frequently leads to a feeling of oppression in the heart area similar to that of angina-pectoris attacks, to shortness of breath and dizziness, or even to unconsciousness. With a pulse that is nearly nonexistent, the patient is pale and driven. Often, congestion in the lungs and liver occurs, and at the end of the attack one may experience a flood of light- colored urine.

The therapy employed by orthodox medicine once again illuminates the fundamental problem. In addition to the aforementioned administration of sedatives that block emotions from affecting the physical heart, stimulation of the vagus nerve is the primary recommendation. With the activation of the antagonist to the sympathetic nervous system, the heart is also calmed down, meaning the sympathetic nervous system that is responsible for the stimulation and activation of the heart is overruled. This situation becomes particularly clear when heart racing attacks occur at night during sleep. Even if a person no longer remembers it when he wakes up, the stirring probably lies in his dreams and, therefore, in the psychological realm. People affected by this condition are apparently emotionally overstimulated. However, their emotions do not reach their conscious minds at all. Instead of being touched emotionally, they experience the racing movements of the heart; instead of racing feelings they have a racing heart. This is similar to blushing. If a person would admit the association that he has with a certain suggestive joke, his face would not have to transform into a red lantern and, thereby, proclaim the truth to the entire world.

When a person has a heart racing attack, it should be clear to her that the reasons for it lie within. In addition, she should ask herself what is ailing her. In the compulsion that one often feels, the relationship to one's own suppressed instinctive impulses becomes physically comprehensible. The issue of "when" can also be important. One can often learn directly, and almost always symbolically, the reason that causes somebody's blood to boil from the specific triggering situation. The oppressive feeling in the middle of the chest indicates with a wonderful simplicity that something has reached an impasse precisely there.

The psychosomatic nature of dizziness and unconsciousness is obvious. First, someone lies to himself and, when this apparently does not do the trick, he flees into that other world where he is no longer dependent on his unpleasant, honest, conscious mind. Rather, he becomes dizzy and, eventually, unconscious. Naturally, much of the information found in the section about heart racing originating from the sinus node also applies to attack-like tachycardia and, therefore, does not need repeating.

6.4 Extrasystoles—Stumbling Blocks on the Path of the Heart

Extrasystoles are premature heartbeats. An irregular impulse center in the atrium or ventricle area outstrips the sinus node and, with its hasty impulse, deprives it of its power. Then, the balance of power becomes reversed for a short period of time. The heart stumbles because of this unexpected beat and it frequently requires a period of adjustment for the sinus node to get everything under control again. Its next regular impulse puts the heart back on the right track. The patient experiences the extended pause as the heart missing a beat and the next beat as particularly distressing. Both situations trigger the fear that the heart could stop beating completely or that a stroke could hit. As a matter of fact, extrasystoles can be early signs of other forms of cardiac arrhythmia that are much more serious, such as heart flutter and fibrillation. However, occasionally they also occur in people who clinically have a sound heart.

The extrasystoles indicate that a person's center has lost its rhythm. The reason for this can be found in certain uncoordinated behavior patterns of parts of the heart that vehemently refuse to pay tribute to the mutual center. Those who demand more than their share, apparently are unwilling to subject themselves to a higher ideal, insisting on their minority vote. They swim against the stream intentionally and thereby draw attention to themselves. Naturally, this type of behavior is unconscious and only becomes visible because of the honesty of the heart. The reasons for get- ting-out-of-rhythm are numerous and have been researched extensively by the medical profession. They range from basic causes, such as brain operations, to any form of nervousness. An overdose of cerebral stimulants such as adrenaline and caffeine, or medicine containing digitalis, may also cause these problems, as might lack of sleep and excessive intake of nicotine or coffee. The stumbling block can also be an overly full stomach, flatulence or serious disorders such as myocarditis, coronary sclerosis, or even the onset of a heart attack. There is little over which the heart and its owner could not stumble. If the affected individual experiences this stumbling and getting-out-of-rhythm consciously, the heart has nothing to fear. Once again, it is the suppression of the experiences that forces them onto the physical heart.

Therefore, those who suffer from extrasystoles are out of rhythm, without admitting it to themselves. They can only experience it through the heart as it vicariously deviates from its role. The primary learning task is to consciously play the old role one has taken on. If the affected individual was consciously facing her central need to be special and unique, her heart would not have to take her place in the drama and deviate from the norm. In addition, it is important to learn to live one's own individuality, to pursue the path of individuation, meaning nothing more than going one's own way. A part of this path may also be to trespass certain (social) taboos. As long as the affected person consciously experiences this, the heart can remain within the prescribed tracks.

Consciously following the path of individuation is certainly the highest level of this theme, although any type of having one's own way, any desire for something special as well as demonstrative clowning around is healthier in the figurative sense than on the level of the physical heart. Even a person who has nonsense in his heart should not express it through the physical organ since he and his environment will benefit more from it on all other levels. He might threaten to become a buffoon due to the special treatment he expects, at which point it is definitely time to change over to individuality and originality on a higher level. The allopathic concept of conformism only forces the heart to do the most peculiar somersaults and sideways leaps, in order to adhere to the set standards.

The therapy prescribed by orthodox medicine includes many things and excludes little. From a massive dose of cortisone (for myocarditis), to digitalis, to the well-known beta blockers, as well as psychiatric drugs or even antiepileptic drugs—all of these agents have been administered "with success." Professor

Heart-Aches

Klepzig[17], head physician of a clinic for cardiovascular diseases, writes very openly on this topic in his classical book: "It should not be concealed that some patients defy all attempts at treatment and complain of discomfort time and again. In those cases, one should advise them to become accustomed to the disorder rather than paying any particular attention to it." This attitude, typical for orthodox medicine, is naturally in complete harmony with the tendency of the patient to suppress the problems and will not help in their (re)solution. The deeper meaning of the symptom requires exactly the opposite: The patient must learn to feel disturbed and be consciously aware of his "stumbling." He should let each new incidence of stumbling (extrasystole) jar him out of the same old rut emotionally instead of physically. Every time the heart loses its rhythm, the situation is caused by an emotional problem in an area that touches the center of life. Once again, bringing these incidents to the conscious level is the actual concern of the symptom. It affords an opportunity to return to a healthy hierarchy within the heart and, therefore, to the dominion of the holy within one's own center.

6.5 Flutter and Fibrillation

The term atrial flutter refers to periodic, uniform flutter waves with frequencies with between 220 and 370 beats per minute. In the very rare case of 1:1 transmission, there is a ventricle flutter with the same frequency. However, in most of the cases, the ventricles only beat at every second or third beat of the atrium, and the heart rhythm remains regular. An arrhythmia occurs if the ventricles beat with alternating frequencies. If the atrial walls pulsate in an uncoordinated and ineffective manner, and disordered fibrillation waves occur with frequencies between 400 to 700 contractions per minute, the condition is called atrial fibrillation. If the electrical impulses from the atrium strike the heart ventricles too often, the ventricles are no longer able of transport enough blood with sufficient pressure in the brief time available. Therefore, the frequently occurring blockage

The Heart Out of Rhythm

of the transmission from the atria to the ventricles can be an advantage for the heart, preserving its functional capacity.

In this case, the ventricles definitely fall into an absolute arrhythmia. Transitions between atrial flutter and fibrillation may occur and both may be the preliminary stages for corresponding, but incomparably more dangerous, conditions in the ventricles. Atrial flutter and fibrillation also have the same medical causes which, in their diversity, largely correspond to those of the extrasystoles. Circulating impulses in the area of the atrium may enhance this effect again, by finding excitable cells as they return to their starting point.

When this is the case, the affected person must admit that his impulses are spinning circles in relation to the center of his life. If absolute arrhythmia affects him, he can admit to himself that an absolute chaos of information reigns in his center. In concrete terms, this means that the affected individual lives in a situation in which he has all the necessary information but can impose neither order nor hierarchy on it. With the abundance of stimulation, he turns in circles without finding his way out. But above all, he is not conscious of this situation, which is why the condition has manifested in his heart.

A typical example is a patient who, after a decade, still suffers from fixation on her divorce or the financial inequity that accompanies it. Without consciously admitting to herself that her entire life circulates around this theme and that she is not able to tackle anything else, she will touch this topic in every conversation. The world around her is familiar with this pattern to the point of weariness, but the patient still does not recognize it. Instead, she continues to turn in unconscious circles and allows the stimulating impulses to circulate within her heart.

The symptoms correspond to frequent extrasystoles and extend from dizziness, feelings of light-headedness, an undefinable feeling of pressure in the chest, up to a condition resembling angina pectoris. In severe cases, even a loss of consciousness and convulsions similar to those of epilepsy may occur—even a heart attack is possible. However, most patients merely complain of a racing heart.

The interpretation of these symptoms corresponds to those explained above. One additional element is the symptom of fear, already implied by the word flutter. If someone is in a flutter, he is apparently nervous, even afraid. Nerves may flutter as well, in the same way as the heart. Trembling with fear is closely related to those symptoms, a theme that touches the very center of a person. A person whose knees shake is apparently afraid to take a stand. An individual with shaky nerves is afraid of cracking up. However, when the atrium flutters, the fear is already in the vestibule of his heart's temple. One step further, and the center of life is threatened. The idea that "heart flutter" also relates to love and fear can be experienced very nicely in French director Louis Malle's movie of the same title. The light-headedness due to inadequate circulation may be considered an indication that the vital energy is sufficient for the most central areas, but no longer for the periphery. The loss of consciousness emphasizes these circumstances as well. Therefore, both symptoms place the head in a secondary role. Apparently, the blood is necessary for more important things than intellectual games. The vehement restlessness in the heart area illustrates the main stage, on which the struggle for existence is raging, and on which it will be decided. As a frequent complication, an embolism may occur which touches different problematic topics depending on the organ in which it appears: the area of communication for the lungs, control issues for the brain, and the area of movement for the extremities.

As possible treatments, orthodox medicine primarily prefers the approach of electrical defibrillation, in addition to the treatments described for the symptoms of extrasystoles and prophylactic blood liquefaction in the case of embolism. This electrical shock for the heart (described in the chapter on complications of cardiac infarction) almost carries a homeopathic aspect in the way it treats over-stimulation with over-stimulation. Through the overpowering electric impulse, all rebellious impulse centers in the heart are abruptly stopped—hoping that the proper center, or at least a somewhat responsible center, will assume dominance afterwards.

The situation that occurs when the ventricles begin to flutter or fibrillate is similar in principle but considerably more explosive. When flutter occurs, which frequently precedes fibrillation, the blood circulation is strongly reduced. In the case of fibrillation, circulation is completely cut off and death occurs within seconds. The most frequent physical cause for this is the infarct. However, medical science with its heart catheterization and heart surgery is also among the immediate triggers, as well as accidents with electricity, myocarditis, and severe heart failure. At the open heart, the flutter can be seen as a surging or agitation similar to a raging hurricane. This is the death struggle of a heart that really is destined to die without outside help.

In their brutal directness, the acute measures taken by orthodox medicine once again show a large degree of honesty. In the case of fibrillation, corresponding to an acute cardiac arrest, it recommends punching the patient a number of times vigorously in the heart area. According to Klepzig, such blows have already saved lives on many occasions. Those vigorous punches very directly mark the area that is of sole importance. They also convey a clear message: time has come to wake up to life, to finally get one's act together, and to decide on *one* impulse center and *one* goal, namely, to live. All other measures, especially defibrillation, use this violent approach. The injection of local anesthetic into the middle of the heart is nothing more than a stab into the heart followed by the anesthetization of the panicking impulse centers.

Finally, heart massage and mouth-to-mouth resuscitation are also recommended. However, those are not really therapeutic measures but follow the objective of winning time by helping the organism to perform those tasks it no longer has the ability to accomplish voluntarily. The massaging hands simply ignore the electrical chaos within the heart and imitate its pumping movements, though with a trace of violence. For old people, it is sometimes even necessary to break ribs which have lost their elasticity. Artificial respiration aims in the same direction, since it forces the victim to participate in a form of communication that the patient already discontinued.

It is important to be cautious when interpreting this and other terminal states, although every state is open to interpretation. In this sense, heart failure could be interpreted as a central subordinate failure that remained unconscious. Consequently, heart failure would be a totally unconscious death, and the dying person practically a "failure" in terms of his main theme in life. However, a human being is bound to die and, therefore, to find a way to do so. Ultimately, it is time to renounce this world and, thereby, to renounce life itself. Renouncing life can be a very conscious step, a step that leads back to one's own soul center and so, once again, to become one. Therefore, the overexcited condition of heart fibrillation may be focused on the task of finding a way out of the existing chaos. This last act, crossing over the gulf between life and death, could be the challenge of the moment. Then, on the other side, true peace awaits the soul; the soul find its proverbial eternal peace. The interpretation of such a situation is superfluous, since only the one who has become directly involved can decide what is of paramount importance for him and his departure. However, at that very moment, he is usually concerned with more important tasks than conveying information on this matter to others.

6.6 Mechanical Block Busters

Several different forms of heart block, blockage of the stimulus conduction within the heart, are known. The ones that are most important relate to the connection of the sinus node with the atrioventricular node, the so-called atrioventricular asequences or atrioventricular blocks. Heart block is classified by degree and in the case of a first-degree heart block, the ventricular activation time between the atrium and the ventricle is merely extended. This disorder does not create any symptoms.

The Heart Out of Rhythm

It can be an early sign of a serious heart disorder, but it also surfaces in a heart that is clinically healthy. However, when the patient receives the information about this diagnosis after an ECG examination, he should ask himself whether he might be quite slow in understanding matters of the heart. Apparently, it takes more time than planned for the most important messages to spread within his inner center.

The most frequent disorder is a second-degree heart block. In this situation, electric impulses take longer to reach the ventricles with each beat, until finally one ventricle contraction is completely skipped. This usually develops into a third-degree heart block, where no impulses reach the ventricles from the atria which, therefore, beat with their own intrinsic rhythm. While the person suffering from the second-degree heart block must admit to himself that he is extremely slow to catch on, only the perception that the connection to his heart has completely disengaged will help the patient with third-degree heart block. Two masters rule over his center. Both are independent of each other, wherein the work performed by the weaker ruler of the atria has become completely senseless. The physical heart proves the wisdom of the Bible that one heart cannot serve two masters. The frequency of the atria, that usually tends to be around eighty beats per minute, is no longer of any use to the heart. The frequency of the ventricles, around forty beats per minute, is too low to maintain the circulation adequately. Such a substitute rhythm, that can sometimes even sink to twenty beats per minute, ultimately only permits a substitute life. As a result of the extremely slow beat of the ventricles, the cardiac output, the flow of blood, sinks beneath critical levels and, in addition to symptoms such as heart pressure and loss of consciousness, convulsive fits may occur if the heart beat drops below twenty beats per minute.

These convulsive conditions, similar to epilepsy and so-called Adams-Stokes seizures, are caused by an inadequate supply of oxygen to the brain. Convulsions generally indicate a frustrating struggle within an area of the body that is in a desperate situation. The muscular cramp in the calf after a long soccer game, for example, makes it clear that one has reached the threshold of pain for the muscles. In this condition, all further efforts only create a futile spasmodic state and no performance. In the convulsive state, the affected areas constrict themselves. They close up, as if they wanted to express: "Things cannot go on like this—at least not with me." A cramp is an expression of a struggle; in this special case, it is a true work stoppage. If one does not fulfill the conditions of the body for a better supply of oxygen and nutrients, soon nothing will function any longer. Such strikes within the body are almost always won by the parts on strike. However, the heart is responsible enough to ensure that strikes occur only in the most extreme emergencies. The brain also persistently asserts itself with its strike conditions. Worst case, the patient must remain constantly in the horizontal position, in order to guarantee an adequate supply of blood to the brain.

The insufficient output of blood very quickly leads to an enlargement of the heart and stroke-volume hypertension. Both can increase the tendency towards cardiac insufficiency. A heart with a total heart block and complete arrhythmia nearly always has been damaged previously, usually through constriction and hardening of the coronary vessels, which can also happen in rare cases when the heart muscle suffers severe damage in the course of myocarditis.

From the clinical perspective, the afflicted one should understand that he has gone too far with the themes of the heart or that things are now out of hand. Every attempt for order and organization in his heart has failed due to theses blocks. He is no longer capable of providing a rhythm for his center and his life. The absolute arrhythmia is an expression of the absolute chaos at the center of his life. Valid standards or any obligatory tempo no longer exist. All that remains is anarchy. Rudolf Steiner's theory that all life is rhythm elucidates how closely this condition approaches one's lethal end. If he is correct, life is facing its last moments.

The Heart Out of Rhythm

The therapy prescribed by orthodox medicine is once again quite illuminating. Since every subsequent attack could be the last, there is no question about massive intervention and equipping the patient with a pacemaker. This sounds routine and, indeed, has become routine today. Thousands of patients have a mechanical pacemaker installed every year. Even the language reveals that this is a very odd form of therapy to say the least. Usually, one replaces spare parts in cars or other machines. As usual, medical science hides this very fact by using a Latin word and "implants" the pacemaker. But what type of "plant" is planted under the skin in such a routine manner?

Technically, a pacemaker is an electrical device, that causes the heart to beat by releasing electrical discharges. It is sewn in under the chest muscle, and supplies the heart with its impulses through a catheter that has been pushed into the heart. With this small machine, medical science is able to put an end to the chaos within the heart and to induce a reliable, stable rhythm. Although without doubt one can overcome chaos because the pacemaker easily dominates its organic competition within the heart, the rhythm provided by the pacemaker may cause problems. Strictly speaking, the pacemaker cannot supply a rhythm but merely beats the time mechanically.

This puts the entire exchange into a very honest perspective: as much as a the rhythm resonates with life, simply beating time belongs to the world of lifeless machines. The original ability to adapt to the ups and downs of life and his emotions is now dominated by a machine, one which naturally beats its time quite independent of any emotions and feelings. The flexibility of life has been replaced by the strict and reliable standard of a machine. The affected individual is safe from the unpredictability of his heart with its leaps and skips, but also from real life. Everything alive has a rhythm, but only the world of lifeless machines is bound to a strict beat. With the little robot that helps the heart to its feet, which carries out its monotonous activities to gain survival, medical science has succeeded in introducing a true strikebreaker. It prevents all possible convulsive attacks of the brain, but also all joyful leaps of the heart. Instead of lively harmony, a calculated and predictable reliability set by the surgeon is now in charge. In a world that places these values above almost everything else, the affected person may not even notice that life is something more than just survival.

In such a situation, it would be honest to deal with the issue of death founded by the dead clock within one's own chest. In this manner, it is possible to perceive how many dead and machine-like elements have already taken possession of one's life. The enormous fear of the incalculable movements within the living center has apparently triumphed. However, with the machine's power within the heart, not only has fear disappeared, but one of the primary qualities of life has vanished as well. Precisely due to awareness of this outcome, it may be possible to see through all the things that are dead and withdrawn from life that have settled in the heart; at the same time it may grant recognition to them. If we use music as our reference point and consider rhythm and beat to be two necessary but opposite poles, an image emerges that also applies to the heart. Rhythm is the individual spirit—lively and sometimes overly rambunctious—that lends its uniqueness to a piece of music and to life. In contrast, the beat provides necessary order and measure. Beat without rhythm takes on a quality that is hostile to life because of its rigidity and ultimate lifeless quality. However rhythm without a beat is also hostile to life; it is chaotic and boundless.

Consequently, a person who has an implanted pacemaker as a result of massive rhythmic disorders should admit to himself that to date he has lived too little of his own special characteristics and individuality. At this point, his heart had to jump into the breach. Also when the overstrain on the heart threatened to end in failure, the pacemaker was an honest rescue attempt, exemplifying how much proper measure and machinelike adaptation and reliability have displaced the importance of one's own liveliness. Now, the machine rules a living, rhythmic organ—the heart.

The Heart Out of Rhythm

Even more often, a pacemaker is implanted when the heart is no longer capable of generating the necessary frequency. Modem pacemakers only provide a beat when one is necessary—when the frequency falls below life-threatening levels. As a result, their owners are less dependent upon the machine and the pacemaker is delegated to the role of a safety net that prevents the recipient from fleeing into the hereafter—into eternal peace—at the first opportunity.

7.

Cardiac Insufficiency—The Failing Heart

When the heart is no longer capable of fully transporting the venous blood supply to the arteries, a backup occurs. This results in cardiac insufficiency; that is, in *congestive heart failure*. Expressed in simpler terms, the heart can no longer cope with its work. This condition usually develops slowly and only becomes acute in very strenuous situations, such as operations, fever attacks, or physical exertion. In these cases, the term *tolerance insufficiency* is used. Left untreated, this condition gradually develops into *insufficiency at rest,* in which signs of heart failure occur even while the patient is resting. Its clinical causes range from inadequate circulation (which may, in turn, be caused by coronary arteriosclerosis) to poisoning and excessively high blood pressure. Valvular defects can also be a cause, as well as pericardial effusion and arrhythmia, either from atrioventricular block, ventricle flutter, or fibrillation.

As a direct result of heart failure, the circulatory flow falls below its required level, causing the body's tissues to receive an inadequate supply of blood. Having overdrawn all available oxygen from the blood, these tissues tend to turn blue, a condition known as *cyanosis*. This effect is especially conspicuous

Cardiac Insufficiency—The Failing Heart

when there is a respiratory obstruction due to pulmonary congestion, as in the case of left ventricular failure. The backup of blood occurring outside the heart results in an increase of pressure in the veins. In this life-threatening condition, the organism attempts to correct the problem with all the means available. When a decrease in blood pressure is registered by the pressure receptors, the sympathetic nervous system is put in a state of alarm. The nerves and hormones spring into action, thus increasing the force of myocardial contraction and the frequency of the heart beat. The blood vessels constrict, which raises blood pressure. Through the narrowing of the veins, and resultant increase in venous pressure, the heart is filled more adequately, thereby increasing the force of myocardial contraction. In addition, constriction of the kidney vessels causes fluid to be withheld, increasing both the volume and pressure of the blood. In order to transport more oxygen under these conditions, the number of red blood corpuscles increases, a condition called *polyglobulism*.

If the heart is still capable of reacting positively to stimuli, all these interrelated effects become focused on a single goal: that the heart accept the challenge and pull itself together again. Otherwise, the opposite occurs. Stimulation of the sympathetic nervous system and retention of fluid increase pressure on the heart, as well as in the veins. If the heart can no longer meet these demands, its condition further deteriorates. Likewise, while the increase in red blood corpuscles expands the blood's ability to transport oxygen, it also thickens the blood, making it even more difficult to flow. If myocardial contractions are weakened as a result of the increased amount of blood and elevated pressure, *dilation* (enlargement) of the heart occurs and the muscle fibers are overstretched. This results in a decrease of the contractile force. Fiber ruptures and destruction of muscle cells further intensify the clinical picture. Doctors refer to this as a "stretched- out' heart.

In this desperate condition, the medical profession differentiates between failure of the left and right sides of the heart. Left sided failure usually stems from high blood pressure, failure of the aortic valve, or mitral regurgitation. This can cause respiratory complaints or even pulmonary edema due to backup in the lungs. When fluid has been discharged into the lungs, so-called "cardiac asthma," or *congestive catarrh*, can occur. Alternatively, congestive pneumonia may be caused by infection from the discharged cardiac fluid. Failure of the left side of the heart often causes failure of the right side and, consequently, leads to the failure of both sides. However, failure of the right side can also be caused by a valvular defect in the right side or by mitral stenosis. The primary symptoms are back up of blood into the venous system, enlargement and hardening of the liver, edema in the legs, and effusions in the chest and abdominal cavity. In addition to a pale blue, the patient's face can take on a yellowish hue, indicating liver involvement.

Congestive heart failure most often involves failure of both sides, with the left side failing first. Since the right side is unaccustomed to working alone, it fails very quickly after the left side. Paradoxically, patients may subjectively feel better at the same time as their functional capacity diminishes, since congestion in the lungs and shortness of breath subside simultaneously.

Our interpretation of congestive heart failure becomes obvious when we consider its diagnosis. The Greek word *did* means "through, throughout," while gnosis means "realization." Thus, the meaning of *diagnosis* is "seeing through," or "seeing through the foreground." In this case, the foreground is the failure of the physical heart and the background is the failure of the heart in its figurative sense. When the physical heart can no longer meet the demands placed on it, the resulting symptoms point to the emotional realm. The accomplishments of the heart have earned the rating "unsatisfactory." The basic psychological situation that has led to this dead-end can be distinguished from the physical defects described above. Whether caused by decades of Sisyphean work, damage to the heart valve, or a long battle against the inner resistance of a constricted flow of vital energy (as in the case of high blood pressure), the result is the same: the center

Cardiac Insufficiency—The Failing Heart

of life gives up. In its resignation, the physical heart admits failure in terms of its themes and tasks. The patient, incapable of succeeding in the heart's tasks, surrenders. The patient, however, does not admit this fact to himself. Only the physical heart demands honesty, since everything revolves around it.

The heart also embodies the task to be performed. It expands and stretches both its individual fibers and itself as a whole. However, what is life-threatening on the physical level offers a chance for redemption on the emotional level. One has the opportunity to expand and surpass oneself, and become more open, in the figurative sense, to the flow of vital energy. Only if this inner expansion takes place, can the physical heart be saved from its dramatic expression of this theme and gradually return to its appropriate, narrower boundaries. Openness, expansiveness, and boundlessness are general goals in the realm of human emotions. If these shift to the physical dimension, the body suffers the consequences, at least as long as it is capable of doing so. Heart failure is the point at which the physical limits have been reached, and at which they await their emotional deliverance. Fasting and other types of therapy have proven that even "stretched-out" hearts can regain their shape if inner expansiveness takes place within the heart.

On the other hand, the cautions mentioned in the discussion of fibrillation apply here as well. Heart failure is the most frequent way for life to end. If the heart of an elderly, but otherwise healthy, person stops without any apparent physiological cause, medical science considers this to be heart failure. Life must end at some point and every death certificate requires a diagnosis. As a matter of fact, a determination of cardiac arrest can always be made. In such cases, diagnosis of a heart problem would be superfluous. At most, it could be stated that failure of the physical heart indicated it was time to deny the physical world and renounce one's life within it. The symptoms of heart failure force a patient to rest, to lie down and prepare for the transition into that other life. This change is instigated by the breaking down of the heart. One's bed becomes the last resting place and one's rest becomes the final, and apparently deserved, rest.

During the crisis of heart failure, other pathological processes of secondary importance also reveal their messages. The most common of these is failure of the left ventricle, in which blood becomes congested in the lungs and ultimately triggers pulmonary edema through the discharge of blood serum. In earlier times, many patients suffocated internally, or drowned in their own "emotional water." Water is considered the element most representative of the emotions. In a medical emergency such as this, the emotional element is restrained, a fact that is demonstrated by the body in its naive, pictorial-symbolic manner. The communication area of the lungs, which can no longer be aired out, fills up with the "liquid of the soul" that is not able to find another way out.

The result is failure of the right side of the heart as well, since it is no longer capable of pumping blood through the lungs, which have been transformed into an artificial lake. Blood that has become congested before entering the right side of the heart also creates a problem. This exhausted blood returns to the heart and exerts pressure on it. The heart can no longer deal with the dissipated energy that is trying to reenter it, and thus no longer functions smoothly.

The liver becomes enlarged and hardened as a result of the backed-up flood of emotions. Since the liver symbolizes the meaning of life, the *religio,* it serves as an additional reminder of this theme. In fact, the entire ground on which the philosophy of life is played out comes under physical pressure and, thereby, is also emotionally *suppressed.* Again, the problem and the solution are evident from the same image. That which is so dangerous on the physical level holds the potential to solve the problems at the emotional level. Viewing the body as a model for the emotional realm allows one to direct the flow of emotional energy to the theme of "religio" and the meaning of life. For if the vital force would congest around the meaning of life, hope is in sight.

Cardiac Insufficiency—The Failing Heart

For other patients, different dramas may be embodied in a similar manner. The "water of the soul" can also build up in the legs and feet, indicating that movement and progress are in question. The theme of flexibility is addressed directly, since the feet are literally swollen with importance. Water, the emotional element, becomes entrenched in this area and shows how much it can obstruct progress if it is unable to rise and flow to the heart, where it belongs. Patients are forced to put their legs up as often as possible. This, of course, prevents physical progress since it is a resting position. Hindering the body's motion suggests a shortcoming in the figurative sense as well. Since the patient is forced to adopt an attitude of contemplation, however, the symptom provides an opportunity for discovering her true tasks in life.

An archetypal figure of ancient mythology illustrates the type of people who hide behind such symptoms. Oedipus, translated literally, means "edema foot" or "swollen foot." Before he was abandoned as a small child, his feet were pierced to prevent him from moving forward, and thus subjecting himself to death. However, Oedipus had both the good and bad luck of being rescued and forced to fulfill his fate. Although he became the most clever of human beings and the only one capable of solving the riddle of the Sphinx, he was not able to apply this knowledge to his own issues. He experienced how little the mind achieves if it is not directed toward one's own progress in life. In this myth, the swollen feet indicate how Oedipus' steps were obstructed.

Likewise, with respect to one's learning tasks, the emotions can pour into the physical cavity of the abdomen or lead to effusion within the pulmonary membranes. Ultimately, almost any area can swell and, thereby, draw attention to itself. In the most severe case, insufficiency at rest, the patient can no longer do anything but lie flat, concentrate on the heart, and obey its signs. It becomes clear that there is no way around the heart. If the center is not in order, nothing is in order. All conquered and acquired wealth becomes insignificant if the treasures of the heart have been neglected. At this point, anyone would give his kingdom for a healthy heart. In the end, one must face the fact that a healthy heart cannot be bought, not even for a kingdom.

This was true until recently. Medical science has now apparently outwitted fate. Not only has it learned how to implant pacemakers, but also how to transplant living hearts. This operation, so spectacular several years ago, has become routine in some highly specialized medical centers. Moreover, some particularly zealous organ dealers intend that one be able to buy a new heart, much in the same manner that one can purchase other organs. However, whether or not they were purchased, hearts that have been transplanted cannot even be considered on loan; at best, they are replacements. Just as an old car functions like a new one when its engine has been replaced, a heart transplant patient is meant to function like a newborn, according to the modem mechanistic approach.

However, there is a difference between a car and a human being. While an old car accepts the new engine without resistance and functions without a problem, the ungrateful body of a doomed cardiac patient is not interested in a new heart. To the contrary, it does everything in its power to get rid of the lifesaving organ as quickly as possible. Only with the most sophisticated strategy of suppression is it possible to awkwardly control resistance to the new heart. Even so, this resistance continues for the rest of the patient's life. During all the years he lives with the borrowed heart, his defense system must be kept in check with immunosuppressives. As a result, the life that was renewed is always threatened by infection.

Despite many technically successful heart transplants, no reliable studies have demonstrated how the transplanted heart grows in an unfamiliar chest or how it evolves emotionally. Shouldn't physical rejection be considered an expression of unconscious psychological resistance? I can only leave the question open, since I have had no patients in psychotherapy who have undergone a heart transplantation. However, one might conclude from the above discussion that each human being is intended to deal with his own heart and make sure that it remains in the right spot. In physical terms, the heart belongs in its very own place and fits nobody else as well as it does the original owner. However, in the figurative sense, one cannot give it often enough to other people, animals, nature, the entire world, and God.

Donating one's heart at death may possibly compensate for a rigid withholding of the heart during one's lifetime. Perhaps the person never promised his heart to anyone and did not really give it away either. One might prefer to promise to give one's heart to a stranger at a time one does not believe will ever come. What did not happen during one's life, due to lack of courage or generosity, may occur after the death of the physical body. However, donating one's heart can also represent the continuation of generosity and devotion expressed during one's life. What a gift, to be entrusted with such a heart for a second life!

Ultimately, each person must decide for himself to what extent body and soul will be in harmony with one another. Whoever wishes to give away his heart after death cannot go wrong if, before dying, he realizes that it also would be wise to give it away in the figurative sense. Wonderfully enough, the one act does not preclude the other.

8.

Further Problems That Touch the Heart

8.1 Degeneration of the Heart

This disorder of the heart, which occurs with chronic emaciation (dystrophy), chronic inflammatory diseases, or in old age, should be understood primarily as an accompanying symptom. Anatomically, it usually accompanies the so-called *brown atrophy* of myocardial cells, in which degenerated heart cells acquire a brown discoloration. Degeneration of the fibrous tissue (fibrosis) between muscle cells can also occur. In both cases, myocardial contraction is reduced. If the cells of the heart muscle degenerate, or if their structure is loosened due to fibrous tissue, the function of the heart slackens. The heart threatens to fail in its task of circulating the source of vital energy, the blood, through the body.

The heart, the center of life, degenerates or gives up altogether in accordance with the state of its individual cells. Since the patient is not conscious of this development, the heart must depict its drama on the physical stage. This is exemplified by structural changes that transform the muscle cells of the heart (which are responsible for the heart's contractions) into tissue cells (which serve solely as stand-ins and are also responsible for scar formation). The patient simply holds onto his place in life, without accomplishing any real emotional or spiritual work.

Extreme wasting of the body and other symptoms of physical decline also support this interpretation. For example, chronic inflammations that can no longer be controlled by the body represent conflicts that overpower physical and emotional resistance. Ultimately, old age itself is an indication that the center of life has given up, as an unconscious inner act. Even the change in color of its cells from vital red, the color of love and life energy, to brown, an earthy color that radiates less energy, could be interpreted as evidence of this. The transformation from energetic red to earth-brown illustrates the cyclical path of all physical life. On the emotional level, the task becomes one of being conscious of the overdue metamorphosis; that is, the conscious letting go of the material world and returning to infinity, the homeland of the soul.

8.2 Fatty Degeneration of the Heart

A great many organs, including the liver (which develops into the infamous "fatty liver") are involved in cases of extreme obesity. The heart can also degenerate into a fatty heart. Its function is obstructed by the masses of fatty deposits, especially those around the right ventricle and between the muscle layers. The respiratory movements of the pulmonary lobes are inhibited when the size of the thoracic cavity is reduced by the fat. This may intensify into respiratory insufficiency and, in extreme cases, can develop into the pickwickian syndrome, so-called after the fat boy Pickwick, in Dickens' *Pickwick Papers*. In this case, fatty degeneration leads to hypoventilation (reduced quantity of air entering the lungs). As a result of the insufficient oxygen supply and excess of carbon dioxide in the blood, brief periods of fainting and attacks of cyanosis occur. The heart is burdened even more when pressure increases in the pulmonary artery.

The problem of obesity exists in the foreground, where one "carries weight" in a disadvantageous manner. Almost everyone has a weight problem, not just in terms of physical pounds, but through carrying emotional, intellectual, and social weight. The reasons contributing to excess weight on the physical level can be as varied as the significance of the excess pounds.

In the case of fatty degeneration of the heart, the weight placed on the center is displayed in an awkward manner. The patient does not admit to himself the significance of his heart and its central themes in life. He is probably not even aware that this does not represent genuine weight (significance), but rather unnecessary and superfluous fat. On the external level, it may appear impressive, but in reality it only obstructs life.

Due to the lack of consciousness, once again the entire story is told by the body. The fatty heart is not only larger and weightier, but also well insulated because fat is an excellent material with which to insulate and, thereby, isolate the heart. While, on the physical level, the patient experiences a warm feeling around his heart, on the emotional level he is probably less apt to admit the corresponding desire. The layer of fat isolates in both directions; fewer situations affect the patient from the outside, while less can penetrate to the outside from within. Thus, the heart is like a fortress in the middle of the body, protecting both against attacks and other forms of contact, as well as against inner developments or challenges. At the same time, the surrounding world is protected against emotions that, no longer doing justice to their name ("e-motion"), have ceased to move outward. Nothing can happen to the heart that is *wrapped in cotton wool,* either in the positive sense or the negative. The constricted physical heart makes it clear that the life of the heart, and of the entire organism, is obstructed by these many protective and shielding measures. The hindered functioning of the lungs prevents the possibility of communication. Ultimately, such people have *heavy hearts* as well, which is not very surprising considering their actual weight.

Before the patient can overcome the isolation of the heart, the principles embodied in the symptom must be resolved. The heart in the figurative sense has to be taken more seriously, although it should remain well protected in the process. A certain shielding and gentle treatment of the heart is advisable, as well as a retreat into one's own safe nest. On the emotional level, a plump heart would not be necessary if the patient adopted a cozier attitude toward life. In this way, he is not constantly forced off-center and does not become insecure so easily.

8.3 Wind That Goes to the Heart

Many different cardiac disorders are connected to the so-called Roemheld's syndrome, ranging from clinical syndromes resembling angina pectoris to a constant dull pressure on the heart. The heart is put under pressure not by the blood but by the intestines. Thus, the basic problem is not the heart, but a disturbed digestion. The diaphragm becomes elevated so that it irritates or disturbs the heart's function. It becomes apparent that something is out of order when fumes and gases develop. Instead of peaceful, regulated activity, the intestines turn into a witch's cauldron. They seethe and hiss, boil, and sometimes stink if the unpleasant fumes let off steam through the bottom instead of moving upward against the heart.

Once again, language is tactlessly honest in disclosing the patient's feeling that "something stinks." Instead of regular digestion, a stink is made or, worse yet, the heart is tormented. The poisonous gases go straight to the heart, laying siege to the center of life. One cannot push them out the bottom because that would be too honest; besides, others would immediately notice what was wrong. Instead of directing the problem at others in a roundabout way, out of necessity, one allows one's own heart to be affected. The suffering of such a victim of good manners and poor digestion can be deeply moving since he is physically caught between the narrow boundaries of his environment and the vilest gas one can imagine.

Heart-Aches

The basic emotion in this condition is clear. Whatever the patient takes to heart cannot be digested. Since he is not conscious of the situation, the body acts it out for him and performs the drama with its own means. In the process, it becomes clear how strongly the patient believes that things smell. Instead of admitting to himself that he cannot escape from the theme any longer, he pushes it even further away from himself. No one, not even he himself, can be bothered by the vile exhaust fumes that he no longer dares to let out from behind. Instead, he attempts to hide them within himself. But, as is often the case with toxic waste, the furthest dumping grounds are precisely the ones that are most hazardous. What no one else is meant to hear or smell must be felt by the person in his heart.

At the same time, the symptoms indicate which path the release should take. Apparently, the patient has something weighing on his heart. He should admit this to himself. If he would just relax a little and allow the gas to leak out from behind, he would realize that he is under such excessive pressure that he is tense enough to burst. The tense, hard belly that is concealed within his soft body parts speaks the same language. In an unobserved moment, he could also smell just how much he feels that everything stinks. Even the relief for his oppressed heart that he experiences when he does let off steam, illustrates the issue at hand. Once in a while, he should let off steam, in keeping with the old Bavarian saying "if you fart, you have a healthy heart." Initially, such *expression* is required in the concrete sense. It is all the more necessary in the figurative sense because that is the only way to achieve long-term relief. The patient should also admit his tendency to act mainly from behind. In the long run, face-to-face conversations would be more relaxing and eliminate his need to swallow what he cannot later digest. Instead of sitting on his stink bombs, it would do his health more good to throw them. In the case of his career, which is of less interest to the team of body and soul, this may not apply, although careers are not promoted by "sitting" on one's problems. Few things are successfully tackled from behind, either by *making a stink* or by *ass-kissing*. The upper frontal entrance is better suited for dealing with mental-emotional conflicts, while the back is better suited for the physical digestive processes.

9.

Cardiac Neurosis—
Fear of the Heart

While organic heart disease patients lack consciousness of their problems, cardiac neurosis patients are overly conscious. Classical heart-attack patients tend to play down their symptoms, while complaints are complaints in the truest sense of the word for the cardiac neurotic. At every opportunity, such a patient complains about the pain that makes his life so difficult. Although the theme has been perceived clearly, it has been related to the body in a one-sided manner. In general, problems are created within the body; this problem, however, is not embodied but rather projected onto the body. Cardiac neurosis does not use the body as a stage, as do other symptoms, but merely as a projection screen. Although the movie is visible on the screen, its themes cannot be distinguished by analyzing the structure of the screen. In a drama, one watches the depicted problems on the screen, even though they are not actually located there. The cardiac neurotic finds himself in the desperate situation of a movie spectator who, after watching a drama, believes the screen has suffered terrible torments. No matter how many specialists he convinces to examine the screen, they will find no trace of the pain. Still, it would be wrong to presume that the movie spectator imagined everything. In fact, he is right because there actually was horrible pain on the screen. He has certainly perceived it, as clearly as the cardiac neurotic has suffered pain. It is simply a case of confusing the levels.

In such cases, any attempts at medical therapy make the confusion between levels even more evident. It is as unlikely for a symptom to originate in the body as it is for a play to be created on the stage rather than in the playwright or director's mind. Physical symptoms can be compared with a play because something concrete occurs on the physical stage. One can also interfere directly on stage by giving new directions to the actors, obstructing them, or influencing them in some other way. In the case of cardiac neurosis, which in this analogy corresponds to a movie, any attempt to influence the screen directly would be absurd and completely ineffective. For example, an attempt to add colors to the screen would not have even the slightest influence on the movie.

The responsible, orthodox medical doctor, after repeatedly examining the heart without result, will reject medical treatment. In the worst case, the doctor confronted with a complaining patient will prescribe psychopharmacological drugs and tranquilizers instead of psychotherapy. In this case, the patient's vision becomes so blurred that he no longer sees the dramatic movie of his suffering as clearly as he did before. This is obviously not true therapy, but merely a cover-up.

How helpless the medical profession is in this situation is illustrated by the fact that, although many sonorous terms exist for the clinical syndrome of cardiac neurosis, no truly effective therapy has been developed for all it diagnoses. As Reimann commented, "The varying terms for this disorder prove how little it has been comprehended." In 1895, Freud provided a detailed treatment of the clinical syndrome, which he called *anxiety neurosis,* and from which he probably suffered himself. In 1956, Brautigam spoke of *heart hypochondria,* and in 1960 Kulenkampff called it *cardiophobia* (heart phobia). In the United States, it lurks in the literature as *functional cardiovascular disease.* During the nineteenth century, such terms as *functional angina pectoris, stimulated heart, hyperkinesis cordis* (hypermotility of the heart) or simply *nervous throbbing of the heart* were used. The descriptions of the corresponding symptoms indicate that cardiac neurosis was involved in each case.

Fortunately for patients, medical science has not yet succeeded in effectively and permanently suppressing the symptoms. The movie of the symptoms that is projected onto the body is significant for the patient. If he is able to see through its projecting nature, this movie can change his life. Like all symptoms, these are honest and instructive. In the foreground is the patient's fear about his heart, and thus his life. His entire life revolves around this fear and, likewise, around his heart.

Attacks of heart throbbing also occur in the foreground. However, with frequencies of one-hundred to one-hundred-and-forty beats per minute, they are usually less violent than those of paroxysmal tachycardia, although they are more painful. The patient feels thrashed by these beats. The threat he feels is reflected in words such as "heart rumbling," "blustering," and "flickering." In view of such emphatic complaints to the doctor and the lack of objective examination results, the medical profession speaks of *hysterical heart throbbing.* Associated with these rapid and violent palpitations, but also independent of them, many patients feel pain in their heart. They complain about being pierced by pain that feels like a knife stab, as well as about continuous burning pain, soreness, and dull, straining pressure. Sometimes the entire left side of the chest is hypersensitive (hyperalgesia). Extrasystoles often occur as well, accompanied at every pause by fear that the heart will stop beating all together. Since it is possible to induce extrasystoles, Richter[18] assumes that they result from the cardiac neurotic's tendency to always expect the worst. Feelings of constriction in the chest and difficulty breathing often occur as well and may be reminiscent of anginose complaints. The patient's spirits are low and his mood may become depressed.

No matter how often the patient and his heart are examined, no pathological results can be ascertained between attacks, although sympathicotropic agitation can be observed during the attacks. No trigger, at least not on the superficial level, can be found for these symptoms, which usually only manifest during intense states of agitation. Apparently, the reason for this lies in the patient's agitation about his heart and the related fear of death. Although it may be difficult to immediately discover all the triggers for cardioneurotic attacks, the initial one is usually easy to find. According to Richter, one can distinguish four main themes:

1. An encounter with illness, death, or accidents related to the heart.
2. Alarming observations about one's own body.
3. Medical diagnoses that wrongly cast a suspicion on the heart. (In these cases, medical science discreetly speaks of "iatrogenic heart disease".)
4. Psychological conflicts.

Equipped with this framework and an understanding of symbols, it is possible to recognize the triggering symbols and situations, even in the case of cardioneurotic attacks that occur at a later time.

The emotional condition of the cardiac neurotic is clearly different from that of patients with other heart diseases. While individuals with type A personalities who have infarction or angina pectoris find it extremely difficult to take it easy and prefer to play down their complaints, cardiac neurotics tend to impose an exaggerated avoidance of strain on themselves. While the type A manager often finds it impossible to limit his work quota, the cardiac neurotic may radically reduce his work output, even when he is not overburdened, because he is afraid of the "manager syndrome." Often, these patients, who no longer feel capable of working, accept drastic curtailments in their quality of life as well as other areas. In an almost grotesque attempt to refrain from anything that could strain the heart or have an agitating effect, they avoid every physical effort, including sexuality "because heart throbbing always occurs during orgasm." As a result of their fear of a heart attack, some no longer have the courage to drive a car while others avoid elevators or swimming in deep water. They skip the most gripping pages in the newspaper because they might excite or strain the heart. They even stop watching live sports broadcasts and suspense movies.

In addition to avoiding strain, these people develop an exaggerated need to cling, whether to parents, partners, or their doctors. Fear of separation plays a major role as well, and patients avoid being alone under any circumstance. As a result, they often make a childlike, dependent impression. They are incapable of tolerating any form of tension with another person, preferring instead to subjugate themselves unconditionally. This often results in symbiotic relationships, in which the person refuses to be without the other for even a moment.

It is not surprising that cardiac neurotics are statistically more likely to marry than is the average person. Cardiac neurotic men may seek a protective mother figure to help safeguard their threatened life. However, their dependence on this mother figure may become so strong that a love-hate relationship develops. On the one hand, the patient cannot exist without the "mother*"; on the other hand, he feels extremely oppressed by this person. These conflicting feelings are also expressed symptomatically. A racing heart, shooting pain, heart pain, increased blood pressure, profuse sweating, and a beet-red face reflect a pattern of attack and flight. Psychotherapy often reveals an inclination toward murder of the overpowering mother figure. The fear of death is also the fear of killing. Both these fears increase the tendency to flee from a life that holds such terrible possibilities. When the patient becomes conscious of his desire to kill, and thus be liberated, he winds up in a classic double-bind situation: If he kills the mother figure, he fears that he will also die because he cannot remain alone. It is time to cut the umbilical cord, as was done afterbirth. The emotional umbilical cord, which supplies and binds at the same time, must be severed.

In addition to exposing the problem, the symptoms reveal the means for its solution. Their aggressive power challenges the patient to fight the battle rather than passively hide. He must actually kill the mother figure, in a figurative sense, to free himself from dependency. Independence and autonomy can only be achieved if he conquers his tendency to cling by waging a heroic struggle within himself The decisive battle must be fought inwardly, since the real dragon lives within his own breast. Only when he *slays* or *stabs* the dragon, and all his regressive tendencies along with it, is the patient free to go his own way. He must follow in the footsteps of Parsival, who conquered his tendency to cling to his mother *Herzeloide* before he began his search for the Holy Grail.

Since this type of situation occurs at an early developmental stage, it is not surprising that cardiac neurotic symptoms also occur early in life. The dragon must be overcome by the second, or at least third, decade of life. If this does not occur on the emotional level, stabbing and beating will continue in the heart. Unlike heart attack patients, the cardiac neurotic still has his whole life ahead of him. However, he must walk the path and discover his identity. Only if he succeeds in doing so can he begin to confront the power of his ego. Up to this point, his heart is protected against physical illness.

The family doctor is sometimes forced to assume the role of the mother figure. He must repeatedly ward off hypochondriac fears with examinations that reveal no physical problems. Since cardiac neurosis makes the helplessness of orthodox medicine so apparent, doctors often have less appreciation for cardiac neurotics than for their other patients. Moreover, hypochondriasis belongs to the shadow of most medical professionals, and no one enjoys being confronted with his own shadow. By necessity, hypochondriasis is an occupational disease among doctors. Because of their medical training, and the fact that everything revolves around the physical symptoms of illness, they become fixated on the body. Illness could be considered their theme in life. Almost every day, they voluntarily go to a hospital or doctor's office. An underlying love-hate relationship, such as one typically has with one's own problems, is likely to develop. Their concern with illness, however, can be lived out within the profession by projecting it onto their patients, thus providing relief for the doctor. Although hypochondriasis tends to triumph during medical students' university years, it usually diminishes during their professional life. Instead of getting on each other's nerves, the doctor and hypochondriac patient should recognize and accept the symbolic aspect of physical conditions. The concern about physical health can then be transferred to the emotional welfare of the patient.

The hypochondriac attitude also explains a characteristic urge to constantly monitor the heart. This can go so far as an intense obsession to control. The patient listens for the finest movement in his heart and registers every irregularity with great consternation. According to the motto "he who seeks will find much," he focuses intently on his heart, although he does so in a physically fixated manner.

The common therapy employed by orthodox medicine consists of repealed physical examinations and accompanying reassurance that the heart is completely healthy. In the worst case, modern, sophisticated methods of diagnosis can turn up a few insignificant deviations. If the doctor cannot refrain from alarming the patient with these symptoms, they may become intensified through medical intervention, as mentioned above. However, the practitioner will generally attempt to convince the patient that his heart is extremely healthy and he will not die in the near future. This has a reassuring effect on the patient each time, but only lasts temporarily. Ultimately, attempting to convince the cardiac neurotic about his lack of grounds for worry is doomed to failure, even though this attempt is justified from the physical standpoint. Statistics attest to the fact that most young cardiac neurotics are less likely to contract an organic heart disease than is the average person of similar age. However, the patient cannot accept this fact because he feels ill, and therefore justified in his complaints. At the same time, because he feels his symptoms physically, it is very difficult to convince the patient that he is ill on the emotional level. One might say that he is caught up in his own movie and rejects the doctor's position that it is "only" a movie and that his complaints are "just psychological," because this viewpoint contradicts his own experience.

In cases of hypochondriasis, both patients and doctors tend to use similar arguments with respect to organic symptoms. Most doctors reject the emotional background for these symptoms be- cause they see that they exist within the body. Furthermore, they cannot measure the emotional level. This represents a refusal to look at the level on which the movie projector stands. The tendency is to cling fearfully to the projection surface as the one certainty. The person refuses to look at the script, while favoring the colorful reflections on the screen.

Instead of trying to talk the patient out of symptoms that are "just psychological" or "imaginary," it would be more meaningful, and even provide relief in the long term, to guide the patient to truly take her symptoms to heart. She would be struck by their meaning, particularly in light of their symbolic depth. The symptoms of cardiac neurosis are simple to interpret because of their directness, and because they can be easily related to their goal, the soul. The fear of cardiac death is completely justifiable. The attitude of expecting the worst is also legitimate since the heart will someday stop forever. The question is not whether it will happen, but when. In this way, the symptoms direct the patient's attention to the theme of death.

Instead of the senseless and false assertion that she does not have to die, it would be more appropriate to encourage the patient to face this theme, which is of such central importance. Apparently, the patient has neglected to confront this until now, or has suppressed the topic of death and killing. It is legitimate to fear for one's own life or that of a symbiotic partner. However, it would be more valuable to detach this fear from a fixation on physical life and transfer it to the emotional level. Since the fear of death is also the fear of extinction, the irrevocable end, this would open up the spiritual dimension. Religion and spirituality reveal that it is a mistake to maintain this fear. Continuing to overlook the emotional and spiritual dimensions of this theme keeps attention limited to the physical screen. As long as the theme is not consciously addressed, the message must be continually depicted anew in the body. Only if it is accepted and worked through will the pressure behind it subside. Once the meaning of the movie has been comprehended, the movie itself becomes superfluous.

Furthermore, her symptoms force the patient to constantly pay attention to her heart. She must listen compulsively to it and obey its most subtle impulses. The patient rearranges her entire life around this task, reducing her activities to the point of an extreme avoidance of strain. Everything revolves around her heart, and it stands at the center of her life. More than anyone else, the cardiac neurotic takes things to heart, relating almost everything to her heart.

In this description, language makes it clear that these reactions can be understood and only need to be transferred to the emotional level. Apparently, the patient has neglected her emotional center without being aware of the situation. The symptoms now force her to make up for what she has failed to do. She must be detained, and the faster she understands what she has failed to do, the faster she will be released from this embarrassing duty. If she insists on avoiding conscious awareness and limiting herself to the mechanical, physical level, it will take a long time before she is free from the burden. On the other hand, if she understands the principle and learns it with body and soul, she can pass through this process faster. If she places her heart at the center of her life, in the figurative sense, and listens to its voice, she can easily live from its fullness and no longer needs to spare herself by exaggerating. In this way, her life becomes more hearty and fulfilled.

The constant compulsion to observe his center and control his heart can also force him into the state of consciousness that is the goal of spiritual seekers. Since constant awareness of the center, the heart, is also the cardiac neurotic's goal in life, only the circumstances have to be changed. Instead of fearful compulsion and shackles to the physical state of the heart, there must be a voluntary reorientation toward the heart as the focus of emotional life. Furthermore, the cardiac neurotic is forced to be completely conscious and aware during moments of pain. He must live in the here and now, which is also a demand of the spiritual path, and represents a transformation from compulsion to spontaneity.

The cardiac neurotic's tendency to cling expresses his fear of not being complete in himself. However, this apprehension is justified. A human being is not complete and whole until he has integrated his shadow with his personality. The shadow is everything that is rejected by his consciousness. Symptoms are aspects of the shadow and, as long as they have not been retrieved and integrated into consciousness, the person will not be whole. Primarily through relationships, people attempt to integrate their shadow and become whole again. This is why a marriage partner is called "the better half," and why a true partnership is so challenging and exhausting. In this respect, cardiac neurotics are on the right path because they concentrate on marriage and holding onto their relationships more than does the average person. However, their mistake lies in confusing the levels. It is not a matter of holding onto a partner in the physical sense, but on the level of the soul. The point is not to avoid confrontations but to seek them. Only in this way can one learn, both from one's own faults and the faults of one's partner, what it is that is lacking and keeps one from becoming whole again.

Those suffering from heart phobia not only fear the destruction of their physical integrity, but also the disintegration of their ego. Again, this fear is justified. If they listen to the warning signs of their symptoms and focus on the heart and soul level instead of the physical, their spiritual development will not be impeded. The goal of this development is the dissolution of the limited, personal ego in the huge ocean of cosmic consciousness. However, before this goal can be achieved, the ego must be found and experienced. In many respects, the message of these symptoms becomes a guide on the path to the heart, which plays such a central role in all religions and especially their esoteric paths.

Heart-Aches

The cardiac neurotic's physical symptoms complete the picture. Why should a human being not be agitated facing such an enormous task? The racing or galloping heart indicates that it is time to get moving. The smashing beats of the heart that cause the patient to fear being struck dead could also announce that his hour has come and it is time to make his move. Is it surprising that these blows seem so crushing and loud, when he has ignored their message for so long? Should he not thank his body for becoming increasingly sensitive and communicating these hints from his innermost center?

All the conditions identified as triggers symbolically remind a person of the most impending and insistent themes. Encounters with illness, accidents, and death point to the finite nature of our stay on earth and to the tasks that must be mastered before our definite end. The alarming observations regarding one's own body push its absolute mortality into the conscious mind. Medical diagnoses, even if incorrect, stimulate this fear as well since the final diagnosis is a certainty: death by cardiac arrest. All types of psychological conflicts can activate all possible emotional themes, but they always demonstrate that what is required to regain wholeness is still lacking. Experiences of separation remind us even more directly that we are only half in this world when our heart remains divided. This may drive the heart into a racing gallop or give it a stab, or it may feel sore or hypersensitive due to these unmastered themes.

The fact that cardiac neurosis can act as protection against organic heart symptoms, and that angina pectoris will rarely develop, even after years of heart phobia with all the symptoms of angina, is only surprising at first glance. The patient is aware of his heart problems and takes them into account all the time—even if only on the physical level, with its limited opportunities for development. This, however, differentiates him from other heart patients who have banished their heart problems from consciousness for a long time, even when these problems manifest in the body, and who would do anything to avoid being reminded of them. The cardiac neurotic is considerably more open to these problems, and attempts—usually in vain—to convince his environment, including his doctors, of their significance. These patients often fight for years to have their symptoms recognized by other people. Apparently these years of attention are good for the heart, because these patients tend to have fewer organic symptoms than do people who ignore the heart because they do not feel it.

This also proves that illness is a path in and of itself. However, it is quite a strenuous one, when considered exclusively in physical terms. The patient can be thankful for his cardiac neurosis, because it provides him with all the hints needed to set his life back in motion and to proceed on the evolutionary path. There is nothing wrong with everything his symptoms force him to do. However, he must voluntarily transfer what he has experienced on the physical level to the level of the soul.

# 10.

Closing Observations on Heart Problems

The example of cardiac neurosis clarifies one thing that applies to all heart problems in general: the patient is forced to listen to his heart once again. One assumes that the patient did not do this voluntarily before. There is a strong suspicion that he trusted another center, the head, thereby neglecting his heart.

Of course, there must be a reason for human beings to have more than one center. For example, the Indian system assumes seven main energy centers, called *chakras*. The heart chakra, Anahata, is the fourth center and is located in the middle of the system. In comparison, the Western system only recognizes three centers, none of which are as well researched. In our common knowledge and mythology theses three centers are firmly anchored : the head, heart, and belly. Various cultures place emphasis on different centers. In Northern countries, the head predominates, which is why one encounters the cool rationalist in those societies. Mediterranean peoples emphasize the heart, which can be seen in their hot-blooded conflicts, bloody feuds of revenge, and turbulent scenes of jealousy, as well as in their distinct love for children. Cultures such as that of Native Americans function primarily from gut feeling, coming from the center of the belly. This is exhibited in a well-developed intuition and close connection with nature.

However, these three traditions reveal the limitation inherent in developing only one center. While the one-sided, rationally oriented person is lacking in heart, and his coldness has a repulsive effect, the individual who feels bound by emotions often lacks the clear, rational function and may appear vague and unclear. Both of these are usually underdeveloped in intuition (having the right presentiment at the right moment about the right path). This is what the Native American has, although he regards the intellectual function as less important, despite its value in confrontations with both Mediterranean and Northern peoples.

Only if the three centers of head, heart, and belly are in harmony with each other, and if their functions of intellect, feeling, and intuition complement one another, is a person well-rounded. The extent of heart problems, therefore, is an exhortation for people of Western industrial societies to come down from their heady heights. The head is only one of three essential centers, just as the intellect is only one of three functions, even if it is an important one. Apparently, the Western world has overemphasized this center and function, neglecting the emotional world of the heart and the kingdom of intuition, our gut feeling. Our lack of intuition is exemplified by the state of our environment, while our neglect of feelings is reflected in the statistics for illness and resulting morbidity. The solution lies in the harmonization of these three areas. This cannot happen by neglecting the head, but requires a courageous step from the arrogance of the head to the (com)passion of the heart. Intuition is most likely to develop out of the connection between the rational mind and the true feelings of the heart.

II.
The Organic Language of the Circulatory System

1.

Structure and Control

In order to understand the circulation and how it works, it is helpful to use the analogy of a municipal water system, with the heart as the waterworks at its center. However, this image is much too narrow. For one, in the circulatory system every pipe is an independent, living being. Second, the abundance of hierarchically ordered cross-connections and monitoring levels reveals the limitations of the comparison. The circulatory system's control mechanism is so complex that it has taken science a long time to understand its main characteristics, and many factors remain unresearched. All this must be kept in mind in attempting to picture this sophisticated structure. Unfortunately, one has to refer to models, and thus is forced to oversimplify.

An initial impression of the wonders of the circulatory system can be gained by considering the dimension of its network, which includes more than 60,000 miles of piping and extends more than two times around the world. The heart, as the center of the body's kingdom, is connected with all the essential structures within its sovereignty. The heart provides nutrition for each individual cell. The vessels are not just simple pipes, but are differentiated in a variety of complicated structures that are adaptable to all the body's needs.

For this reason, medical science speaks of independent organ systems. For example, the artery wall forms a living, tripartite structure. The inner layer is the *intima,* consisting of endothelial tissue. One may imagine this "most intimate" layer as a sophisticated sieve, permitting only those few substances of the blood that are necessary for its own nutrition to pass through. The robust middle layer, the *media,* follows the delicate intima and consists of muscle cells that provide the vessel with its strength and its power to expand or contract. However, the muscle cells alone could not handle the alternations in blood pressure that occur over time. For this purpose, they are supported by an elastic membrane that prevents the wall from rupturing during these changing conditions, and guarantees a substantial degree of flexibility. Finally, the outer layer, the *adventitia,* consists of firm, connective tissue that cushions the muscle layer and protects the entire vessel. On the exterior of this outer layer are more vessels, which are much smaller than the artery and are responsible for its blood supply.

Since every living being must be nourished, virtually every area of the body has blood vessels. Tissues that can afford to be without vessels, such as those in the cornea of the eye, due to its transparency, are nevertheless dependent on nearby vessels. In order to supply all the countless organs, tissues, and cells, the body has conduits of many sizes—from the main artery, which is as thick as a finger, to hair-like capillaries. The expression "hairlike" is, however, a tremendous oversimplification since these capillaries are ten times finer than the average hair. They are so numerous that, despite their inconceivable delicacy, they would cover the surface of a football field if they were spread out. Through the capillaries, the thinnest living pipes, the heart can supply blood to any point in the body.

The structure of the circulatory system can also be visualized as a tree growing out of the heart. This comparison is so appropriate that the medical profession calls it the *vascular tree.* The main trunk is formed by the main artery. Strong branches lead from this point to all major parts of the body, and from there branch off even further. Ultimately, the branching is so fine that the branches can hardly be seen by the naked eye. The finest endings, the capillaries, allow for exchanges of nutrients and other substances to occur. In this respect, they can be compared with the tree's leaves or, more aptly, with its fibrous roots. A closed circuit is formed, with the finest vessels flowing back together after they have provided oxygen and nutrients to the cells, as well as absorbed waste materials. In this way, the venous system, which transports used blood back to the heart, forms a mirror- image of the vascular tree. The two trees stand very close, almost leaning on each other. A nerve trunk of comparable size usually runs parallel to them.

The signature of a tree is imprinted deep within a human being. It also appears in the bronchial tree of the lungs. However, the function of the vascular tree differs in sophistication from the green tree found in nature. On each level, it is finely attuned to its various needs. At the same time, the control system is monitored by the next highest level. This hierarchical principle is strict but not rigid. Messages can travel in both directions. Through the communication system's network, the central headquarters are informed about everything that occurs at all sites, and can adjust decisions according to the information received.

The finest and most researched control level is that of the *precapillary sphincters,* small, circular muscles located in front of the capillaries that, when contracted, can close the capillaries. These are like the nozzle at the end of a garden hose. If the nozzle is wide open, a strong stream results; if the opening is narrow, however, only a weak stream can pass through. The sphincters react in direct response to the needs of the tissues. If a tissue's oxygen saturation falls, the sphincters open and abundant blood flows into the area. If the oxygen level rises, the sphincters gradually narrow and curb the blood supply.

In addition to this short-term adjustment, the tissues can adapt to changing states of demand over the long term. If a lasting increased demand for nutrients (resulting, for example, from regular physical exercise) cannot be satisfied adequately by the

Structure and Control

existing vessels, new vascular paths are formed. Capillarization constantly adapts to these demands; in other words, the body is always in motion, like a large, busy construction site. Throughout a lifetime, it rebuilds and adapts to each new situation. This explains why people who are physically well trained have better reserves and can compensate better in emergencies than people who have not trained. If one of three paths breaks down, it is not as dangerous as when the only supply line stops functioning. In the case of the heart, this can be a matter of life and death.

The kidneys have a role in controlling circulation. An important precondition for the correct functioning of the circulatory system is an adequate blood supply. If the amount of blood is diminished, for example by becoming bogged down in the legs, or if blood loss occurs due to an open wound, the output of the heart also drops. This, in turn, causes a drop in blood pressure. When the blood pressure is low, less blood is pressed through the kidney filter, thus reducing the excretion of water or urine. If the organism again increases its fluids, the blood volume rises as well. In the reverse case, if blood volume is increased (for example, by drinking an excessive amount of water) both cardiac output and blood pressure increase. In this instance, more blood is filtered by the kidneys, more urine is formed, and the excess is then excreted.

Pressoreceptors or *baroreceptors* have direct control over these mechanisms. Located in the walls of the vessels, these are small sensory nerve terminals that respond to changes in pressure. Like the *chemoreceptors* next to them, which measure oxygen concentration, they pass on the measured values to the vasomotor center in the brain. The vasomotor center is subordinate to the higher brain centers, which are responsible for, among other things, emotional influences on the blood pressure.

Commands from above are conveyed through two central parts of the autonomic nervous system, the *sympathetic* (thoracolumbar) system and the *parasympathetic* (craniosacral) system, or *vagus*. These two opponents regulate the nervous control of all organs. The sympathetic system has a stimulating effect on the heart and circulatory system. It raises blood pressure by constricting the vessels, increases the heartbeat and its output, and prepares the organism for an upcoming attack or flight. Its corresponding hormones are adrenaline, also called "stress hormone," and noradrenaline. The vagus, on the other hand, adjusts the organism for rest and regeneration, inhibits the heart, calms down outer activities, and provides for inner relaxation. Its corresponding hormone is acetylcholine.

This summary of circulation control is, of course, oversimplified. Many other factors, such as the hormones aldosterone and angiotensin, have an effect as well. In addition, connections between the various control components branch widely. The circulation is coordinated with the nervous system at various levels, including the spinal cord, before messages can be directed upward to the vasomotor center or other central areas. At the same time, close feedback between the brain and heart exists at all times.

In a state of excitement, all mechanisms work toward the goal of rapidly bringing the body up to high speed, or putting it into a state of alarm. Because of the interplay of hormones and nerves, the blood can be directed through the local sphincters into any area where it is needed at the moment, such as the muscles of the extremities. At the same time, blood flow in organs such as the kidneys, intestines, or liver is curbed. The heart increases its output and blood pressure is raised. In this hierarchy, the heart ranks above the circulatory system. Thus, for example, a permanent rise in blood pressure is accepted for the sake of securing an adequate cardiac output.

2.

The Basic Structure of Blood Pressure

2.1 The Blood—Symbol of Life

Blood pressure, the decisive measure of circulation, arises from the interplay of blood and vessel walls. Blood symbolizes the power of life. Every child knows instinctively that it is a "special juice." If blood flows from even the most harmless of injuries, the child is horrified. No physiological knowledge is required; the symbolism is conveyed directly at a deep level. Ancient peoples sensed that their vital force was contained in every drop of blood. Since geneticists have discovered the information for the entire human being in each drop of blood, even science must agree with this idea. Many ancient cultures, for which this was a natural assumption, used blood for their magical rituals.

Even today, empirical medicine uses drops of blood for diagnosis in such methods as the pendulum and radionics (a vibrational therapy widely used in England). In light of this, the holistic blood- drop diagnosis of Auras-Blank, which assumes that all essential symptoms are clearly portrayed in one drop of the patient's blood, appears less obscure. The uniqueness of each human being can be proven with blood. This makes blood the bearer of our individuality, as well. The medical profession employs this knowledge in blood tests to establish, for example, paternity.

Language has always recognized that the special relationship between family members is based on blood, and emphasizes their deep bonds. From this point of view, it is clear why religions, such as Judaism, strictly reject the consumption of blood, while others, such as Jehovah's Witnesses, prohibit blood transfusions. Language is also aware of the deeper meaning of blood for a person's character and abilities, stating that "it is in the blood of a person." For someone who is hot-blooded, emotional agitation is intense, while cold-blooded people tend to obey their cool, rational minds. Language often uses phrases referring to blood for decisive situations. A blood feud describes the most extreme form of this emotion, and a bloodthirsty person will stop at nothing.

Ultimately, blood is one of the keystones of religious mysteries. Shamanism is familiar with blood brotherhood through the exchange of blood. This has its basis in the concept that two people will remain forever close and blood-related after their blood has intermingled. Modem times have proven the negative side of this ritual to be true: whatever pathogens the two people had in their blood are also shared after the ritual. If they share the suffering, why should they not also share the joy? Perhaps Native Americans are a step ahead of other cultures in this respect.

In the mystical variation of Buddhism, the Vajrayana, it is self-evident that blood carries a figurative meaning. Blood is treated with great care because all demonical beings are believed to be chasing after it, as the Devil is after their souls. Western religions have largely lost such knowledge, which has often degenerated into superstition. Superstition, however, still knows that the Devil has a pact with the soul signed in blood, and believes that vampires and witches are chasing after this exquisite juice because it is the only thing that can extend their sham lives. In this case, as well as in mythology and fairy tales, blood is an expression of the soul's power. In Western esoterics, this notion is supported by alchemy and by the legend of Parsival, in which three drops of blood in the snow show the soul the way home to the castle of the Holy Grail.

In denominational Christianity, the central significance of blood is expressed in the sacrament of Communion. Catholicism emphasizes that the wine is turned into the blood of Christ during the Eucharist. Thus, the priest drinks the blood of the Redeemer. This act of religious cannibalism is based on the mystical idea that the soul is in the blood. Protestants, who are further removed from the magical world of mysteries, only regard the wine as a symbol of Christ's blood. Nevertheless, they place a great deal of value on consuming this symbol on a regular basis in order to, at least symbolically, bear their Redeemer within.

Even those who have no religious attachments and strongly reject all superstitions recognize the symbolic significance of blood. The movie industry favors this effect when portraying horror scenes. A face smeared with blood triggers greater shock than does a broken or unnaturally bent leg. That the blood may result from a harmless cut, while the leg may be severely injured, is irrelevant.

2.2 Vessel Walls—Symbols of Limitation and Resistance

The idea of blood pressure as an expression of the dynamics of our lives originates in the confrontation that occurs when something liquid flows within something solid; that is, between the blood and the boundary-setting vessel walls. The resistance of these omnipresent walls against the flow of vital energy determines its force and speed. Just as the blood represents our being and individuality, the vessel walls represent the resistance we encounter, the boundaries against which we constantly bump on our path in life. As boundaries, they restrict our stream of life while, at the same time, providing direction and guidance. This makes them essential channels for our energy. Boundaries that are too tight, as well as those that are too wide, can obstruct the flow. Exaggerated narrowness can choke it off, while undue expansiveness can permit it to lose pressure and guidance. The parallels on the emotional level are apparent. A life that encounters vehement resistance will become narrow and inanimate. But a life that is not constricted by boundaries, and not challenged by resistance, cannot prove itself and remains vague and without a red thread.

3.

Hypotension—Life Without Tension

Many people are familiar with the problem of low blood pressure, since it regularly occurs when illness is accompanied by a long period of bed rest. A patient who attempts to leave her bed after several days of fever suddenly feels fatigue, both physically and mentally. When attempting to stand up too quickly, the feet may fail to do their duty and the patient may black out. A cold sweat may break out, and dizziness and a feeling of pressure in the head may occur. This condition, which is quite normal after a fever, is the daily experience for a hypotensive patient. Someone with blood-pressure values below 100 mm Hg, continually feels as if she were getting out of a sickbed. Every illness that requires bed rest represents a step backward to an earlier level, with less burden and responsibility. Through this regression, a state of early childhood, in which all wishes were fulfilled, is experienced again for a short time during the illness. Afterward, however, one cannot hide in bed and must face life again. After a few days, the body has generally recovered enough that it is able to again obey its owner. Likewise, one who is inwardly prepared, can easily face life again.

However, the hypotensive patient gets stuck at this point, often struggling to greet each new day. The issue is to face this day and thus, in the symbolic sense, to face life. If the patient does not understand that the real issue is whether or not to take up the struggle for existence, the problem will become submerged in the shadow. In this case, it will be staged on the physical level. Only in the evening, does the hypotensive patient feel better again, having survived the day and with*stood* this little task of life, which symbolically represents the large task of life. All the accompanying symptoms illustrate this unconscious struggle and the unacknowledged fear of it. Through its symptoms, the body honestly admits that the only way the patient feels well is by lying in a horizontal, resting position in which enough blood can flow into the brain and all symptoms disappear. Any type of exertion that requires an upright position has a bad effect. Dizziness shows that the person is fooling herself about something or deceiving herself about her problems. Standing up physically does not correspond to facing oneself inwardly, a discrepancy that is illustrated by the symptom itself. The person is lying to herself about something in her own mind. Her head is not really active, and her will has no chance to do something either. The shoe pinches in exactly the right place: in the form of pressure in the head.

Flight from the responsibility of facing oneself is obvious in the case of fainting spells. The only power that such a person has is the ability to withdraw and become unconscious at any time. In this way, having left the problem for other people to solve, he feels completely exonerated. Material such as this makes film history: caught in an unequivocal situation by her husband, the guilty lady does not even try to defend herself but falls into a dead faint. In this way, she is rid of her problems for the time being. The husband, who was angry, now has a different set of problems on his hands. He must revive the unconscious woman and ensure that enough blood is flowing into her power center. She is put to bed with her legs elevated and her head as low as possible so that more blood can flow to her brain. With a bottle of perfume, cold water, and an abundance of fresh air, he makes sure she can face herself again. After all, what use is the most impressive display of anger or the hottest conflict if the other person withdraws in a cool, refined manner, using a medical safeguard to flee from responsibility? Since illness and its meaning are taboo themes in society, fainting makes for an elegant escape.

In illustrating this theme, the physiological condition is a perfect match for the social situation. No confrontation takes place between the blood, as the vital force, and the boundary-setting resistance of the vessel walls. The vessel walls do not even try to create resistance; rather, they shrink back, letting the blood flow unimpeded. The drama is one of retreat, and it is performed in a dramatic manner. Yielding to the point of flight is preferred to a challenge. In the same way that blood does not find its way back to the heart but remains clogged in the legs, the emotional vital energy remains stuck somewhere in the periphery. Only through confrontation with vessel walls that provide sufficient resistance can blood mobilize enough strength to flow up to the heart and, from there, to the brain. Similarly, in order to climb a mountain, one must accept challenge and resistance, something the patient is unconsciously unwilling to do.

In the case of fainting, the patient's helplessness, while harmless, succeeds in capturing medical attention. Once again, it reveals the truth that the patient is not willing to face himself. When the pretense is over, he is willing to let enough blood flow to his heart again. On the floor, which is a more honest level, he can regain control relatively quickly. Bringing someone down to earth or making him face the facts is meritorious, even if that person experiences pain through the honesty. The pain, after all, mainly affects the emotional level. In physical terms, the act of falling to the floor is usually harmless, since the person is aware of falling in time to protect himself from bodily harm. It provides an opportunity for the patient to interpret his symptoms, even if this proves unpleasant.

In evolutionary terms, the person has difficulty with one of the most important steps in individual and ethnological development: standing up on one's own legs. Anyone who watches a small child struggling to stand up by himself can sympathize with what humanity achieved ages ago with this one step. Standing upright is also the prerequisite for a sense of uprightness. A person who, as an adult, still has to struggle to stand on his own two feet will also have a corresponding problem with independence. The ability to be independent, to face oneself, and to show steadfastness when necessary, is the prerequisite for any form of personal progress. Someone who cannot stand on two feet, who lies down instead at every opportunity, will not progress in life. Instead of the world lying at his feet, he lies at the feet of the world. And most often, he does not even express humility in this act, which would promote development, but is striving against destiny.

How sensitive some people are is evident in the clinical syndrome of a hyperreactive carotid sinus. The carotid sinus is a spot at the side of the neck from which the vagus can be activated, thereby calming the heart and circulatory system. In people who are hypersensitive, turning or inclining the head can lead to collapse. Even a small movement of the head is more than they can tolerate. If this movement is made abruptly, the soul intervenes immediately, indicating that it can no longer keep up.

All the other accompanying symptoms illustrate and enrich the same central theme. The conspicuous paleness of the skin shows that the patient no longer uses his vital force to its limit. The skin, the outermost zone of the body, is not animated. The antiquated expression "noble paleness" indicates that in earlier times this degree of animation was not proper among high-society women, who were expected to remain withdrawn and far away from "real" life.

Using the analogy of a country, this symbolizes a situation in which the frontier posts are not occupied and no one lives near the border. Thus, powers from beyond the border have an open invitation to penetrate the territory and establish foreign rule over it. Hypotensive patients are constantly threatened by such a danger, because they are incapable of protecting themselves against infringement. Their only defense is passive resistance in the form of civil disobedience, inner emigration, or—the most blatant form—fainting. Another image is that of a snail, which, hiding deep within its shell, may be perceived as hostile by the surrounding world. In its voluntary isolation, the snail does not even stretch out its feelers, but rather pretends not to be at home. It is not surprising that people who have chosen this manner of living are often treated in a demeaning manner. They overlook the fact that they were the ones who first behaved like snails.

One reason that a country does not populate its borderland is fear of the dangers lurking beyond its borders. Likewise, in the hypotensive patient, the so-called "border regions" are inadequate supplied. Lifeless coolness is evident not only in the facial skin with its noble paleness, but also in the skin of the feet and other areas that are devoid of warm, vital energy. This symptom, in itself unpleasant, reveals a deeper meaning that is equally unpleasant. People who get cold feet often have chills going down their backs; both symptoms indicate fear as well as poor circulation in the skin. Someone who always has cold feet lives in constant, unacknowledged fear of life. If a cold sweat breaks out as well, this feeling is intensified, both physically and emotionally.

Cold, undersupplied feet also show how lifeless and inadequate one's contact with the earth is. In this case, the very foundation of one's life is disturbed and it is not easy to find a healthy *standpoint* or get a firm hold. According to these symptoms, stability and steadfastness are a problem. If the patient takes an honest view of the situation, he will probably realize he has already fallen to the ground, and may even have shattered. Thus, he has been defeated before his life struggle could even begin. Someone whose dizziness prevents him from standing upright will also get cold feet before he can face the battle.

The inadequate circulation in cold hands is another truth-telling sign that indicates life is lacking. The constriction of the vessels also reveals fear, the twin brother of narrowness. If a cold hand is extended to greet us, we quickly perceive that it is not a warm welcome. The fact that the person often tries to prove the opposite with his words, and sometimes even apologizes for his cold hands, only shows how embarrassing the honesty of one's hands can be. Deep within, such people are unwilling to make contact. This is even more apparent when sweat, another sign of fear, appears as well. The person who is offered a sweaty hand, that literally slips and slides away, feels rejected rather than accepted. Such a handshake cannot impart any heartiness because it does not come from the heart. The vital force of people with sweaty hands has been withdrawn, revealing through this symptom their constant fear of contact.

Such a handshake often also lacks pressure. The person who is offered a slack, moist, and cool hand feels how little the owner believes in the gesture of welcome. If a person so easily gives his hand to others without resistance, he should not wonder that he often feels he is in someone else's clutches. A hypertensive patient will give this hand a good squeeze. However, it can be quite humorous when two hypotensive hands greet one another simply because convention demands this gesture. They do it, yet they reveal how little control they have over themselves or their lives. Cold, lifeless hands indicate how removed they are from *handling* their own lives and how incapable they are of taking action. In order to take one's life into one's own hands, one must be alive.

The genital organs of both sexes are also strongly dependent on blood pressure. This is particularly evident with the penis. The chronic slackness of the hypotensive patient may be the origin for the expression "jellyfish," which is used when someone fails to stand up for himself or confront a situation. Sexuality, with all its lustful swellings and secretions, depends upon the circulation. Those who are frugal in their circulation tend to fail more often in matters of sexuality, and will never achieve much success in this field.

One symptom that often occurs in connection with low blood pressure, and also carries a similar symbolism, is anemia, the lack of red blood corpuscles. In this case, the blood contains too few of these tiny, flying-saucer shaped transport cells. Their task is to convey the external energy that we encounter in the form of air, prana, vital force, or—scientifically speaking—oxygen, to the body's cells. If there are too few of these cells, the blood stream cannot transport enough vital energy. Accordingly, the patient feels weak. The vital juice is too thin, contains too little substance, and thus is unable to take in the necessary energy and transform it into any type of initiative. The emotional inability to open up to the vital force and make use of it is unconscious but becomes evident through physical, as well as psychological, sluggishness.

The most common medical basis for anemia is iron deficiency. Responsible for the binding of oxygen in the red blood corpuscles, iron initially allows oxygen to be absorbed from the air. In symbolic terms, iron is connected with Mars, the Roman God of War, and his archetypal principle. His warriors are as hard as iron. With their steely fists, iron armor, and violent weapons, they will stop at nothing to conquer the world. Their color is red, like that of iron ore, blood, fire, and energy. Patients suffering from anemia lack this principle, which governs aggression as well as any form of new beginning. If this situation is not experienced consciously, it must be lived out in the shadow. In practical terms, this could be through iron deficiency. The therapy applied by orthodox medicine involves administering an injection of iron into the blood, which demonstrates the problem more clearly than it solves it. Since the patient is not prepared to open up to this principle, administration of iron tends to cause diarrhea (again emphasizing that the patient is "scared shitless") or nausea, rather than simply filling up the iron reserves. In symbolic terms, external violence, in the form of a steel needle, is used to pierce through the skin. This is a thoroughly Mars-like act, since the patient is "raped" into a more Mars-like state of activity.

Medical doctors often attempt to comfort patients by commenting how little can be done to change their constitution and heredity. While this may be correct, it prevents the patient from taking responsibility. It is easier to blame one's constant weakness on constitution, heredity, or an unjust fate. But little can be changed by deferring responsibility or blaming others ("I inherited this from my father..."). This only makes it more difficult to stand on one's own two feet. Even one's own constitution represents a task that must be tackled, especially if it shows these types of symptoms.

4.

Weakness of the Connective Tissue Varicose Veins— Thrombosis

Weakness of the connective tissue with a tendency toward varicose veins, vascular ruptures with resulting thrombosis, and varicose ulcers all belong to the constitution of a hypotensive patient. Connective tissue is the most common material in the body, connecting the organ cells and giving the organs and other body parts their external form. In addition to its connective and formative function, it fulfills the task of giving support. Without connective tissue cells, for example, liver cells that fulfill such tasks as protein synthesis and detoxification would be unable to accomplish the liver's function. Our face, as welt, receives its individual expression through fatty tissue, a form of connective tissue. A lack of firmness in the connective tissue reflects an inability to bond in relationships. Unreliability and an aversion to commitment can also be assumed. Such people usually have few contacts and find it hard to establish relationships. For this reason, they frequently cling to a single relationship, in which they try to find the security they lack within themselves.

Heart-Aches

A lack of stability becomes tangible through the lack of firmness in the body. On such people, tissue hangs like clothing on a rack. This is particularly evident with female breasts, the buttocks, and sometimes the face. Those who let themselves "hang," but do not admit it, cannot avoid being confronted with this fact in the mirror. Although it may be difficult, this is their only chance for honesty. Individual body parts emphasize specific problems that stand out from the overall situation. Someone who lets his buttocks hang has a problem with his power to assert himself. Hanging breasts, however, come naturally with a certain size and require no further interpretation. Something heavy that extends into empty space is bound to hang. However, when slackness rather than weight itself is in the foreground, it may represent neglect in the areas of femininity and nurturing.

Hanging tissue in the face expresses more clearly than could be said in words that a person has resigned himself *faced with life*. Hanging corners of the mouth reveal a deeply etched sullenness. Hanging cheeks indicate a limp person with a doglike expression. Bags under the eyes show both resigned sadness and the uncried tears that such a person carries around. Inner instability is also apparent in the facial features that such a person cannot bear to be exposed to so much honesty. Surgeons are hired to lift in secrecy what the person can no longer carry himself.

Since the formative aspect of the connective tissue is involved, and the patient is visibly not in good form, there must be a corresponding problem on the emotional level. In fact, these people cannot give form to their mental, emotional, and spiritual tasks. They are unable to shape their own environment, instead giving in and allowing themselves to be formed. Usually, this is compounded by a sense of powerlessness and an inability to act. People with weakness in the connective tissue are typical victims. They are wax in the hands of those who are more assertive, to whom they cling, or lean upon, in search of protection.

The fact that it is not so easy for such people to play the victim is revealed by their tissues, which expose a distinct sensitivity and vulnerability that they prefer to consciously deny. People with weakness in the connective tissue are careful not to cause offense or attract attention. Any little shove is immediately documented by the honest body in the form of a bruise. Even a slight offense, in the figurative sense, can cause deep injury. In addition to a high degree of impressionability, there is a tendency to feel resentful and even insulted. It takes time to heal a bruise on the body, not to mention a bruise of the soul. Sometimes an external impact is not necessary, and the small vessels burst on their own. The resulting pattern, called *spider-burst veins,* is visible on the legs of these patients. If they had flawless legs, such patients would feign flexibility and steadfastness, as well as firmness of character, to say nothing of their willingness to make progress. However, the honest colored pencil of the shadow shows up at the most inopportune time. Even plastic surgeons cannot erase these messages from within that are so vexing to the patient.

If the larger vessels draw patterns on the legs, the situation can get even worse. Inflammation of the deep leg veins, general vascular weakness, or infirmity of the embedded connective tissue can induce the blood to meander in leisurely loops instead of purposefully returning to the heart. This causes an overburdening of the venous valves, which correspond in function to the valves of the heart. Normally, they ensure that the blood flows forward toward the heart, and that it never flows backward. However, if the veins are overstretched, the life stream turns away from the heart at a certain phase. A Sisyphean situation, similar to insufficiency of the cardiac valve, in which pressure is extremely lacking, occurs. Doctors speak of *varicose veins,* and patients complain of heavy legs and cramps at night.

Normally, through movement in the deep leg veins and pulsation of the neighboring arteries, the blood is transported slowly but surely in the direction of the heart. Since someone with weakness of the connective tissue usually also has hypotension, too little movement takes place in the arteries and veins of the legs. In both the concrete and figurative sense, there is too much standstill and too little movement. The vital force, which has been sent out sluggishly, returns even more sluggishly and inadequately. Blood congestion occurs mainly in the lower legs, but can also occur in the feet and thighs. The lower legs, in particular, emphasize jumping and moving forward with the corresponding themes. Once again, the issue is ultimately inner movement that symbolically leaves its mark on the external site. The person's vital stream, and thus entire life, develops sluggishly and turns in circles, instead of purposefully moving forward. At times, things can even go backward.

The physical consequences range from edema and cramps to inflammations of the veins and varicose ulcers. Due to congestion in the veins and the reversed direction of blood flow, leakage of fluid may occur in the lower legs and feet. When the blood becomes bogged down in the tissues, the emotional element, symbolized by water, is no longer in motion and becomes congested. As a result, the circulation becomes centered in the lower half of the body, emphasizing this area. The legs feel so heavy that the patient can hardly carry them. Heaviness and the sense of being earthbound are reflections of the person's emotional state. Instead of elasticity and flexibility, sluggishness and brittleness predominate. This cannot be mistaken for good relaxation, but rather is a cramp. Particularly at night, these cramps try to force the patient *to find his feet.* The fact that they occur mainly at night indicates that their emotional, rather than physical, basis. Like the symptoms of the body, dreams also express the shadow, which is not permitted to enter the conscious mind during the day time.

Edema gradually causes the border areas, which already have poor circulation, to atrophy. The skin loses its elasticity and adaptability, literally becoming thinner. A minor injury or inflammation is then sufficient to cause an ulcer to form on the lower leg. Varicose ulcers are not in themselves dangerous, but are extremely bothersome and a widespread, chronic symptom of aging. The skin, which has been neglected and under supplied for a long time, collapses. As in the case of the country that has not settled its borders, the patient reaches a point where his borders have been opened, albeit violently. The water of life has crossed the borders, and all possible pathogens can happily enter the country. This is actually therapy for the body because everything that has been fearfully locked inside can leave, even if only on the physical level.

In therapeutic terms, the patient must now be concerned with his skin. At least on a physical level, it is clear how thin and sensitive this boundary layer is. Every day the patient must take care of his open wounds and replace the collapsed skin with carefully wrapped bandages. This maintenance of the border, better late than never, is a challenging task. Changing the bandage everyday is likely to briefly reopen the wound. After months of suffering open wounds and increased sensitivity, the patient is likely to admit that he is quite thin skinned.

It is not surprising that many patients take poor care of their varicose ulcers. It appears that such patients need these outlets for the sake of detoxification. In fact, this is supported by the claims of many naturopaths. It is considered a sign of progress if all the poison that has backed up in the soul during times of giving in and yielding is now eliminated, at least symbolically, through the legs. In this respect, naturopaths are completely right. Orthodox members of the medical profession who have not been able to find any toxins in the excretions are correct as well, since it is a symbolic detoxification. Patients need their varicose ulcers because these are the only openings they have. Of course, the solution is only temporary, but it is better than no openness at all.

Inflammation of the veins (thrombophlebitis) is often associated with ulcers of the lower leg. Its worst form is inflammatory thrombosis of the deep leg veins, which drives more blood into the superficial veins. In such cases, congestion and excessive strain occur on a regular basis, and embolism may develop at a deeper level. When the superficial inflammation of venous thrombosis leads to the development of ulcers in the lower legs, patients can find themselves in a vicious cycle. On the physical level, slowing of the blood flow is the most essential prerequisite for venous thrombosis, which can develop after a period of forced physical rest, such as after an operation or any other long period of bed rest. At the same time, because this is precisely the type of "emergency exit" that patients tend to take, their reaction to their symptoms can actually drive them deeper into those symptoms. Varicose veins are another condition that promotes inflammation of the veins while simultaneously being promoted by that inflammation.

Although the situation grows increasingly hopeless, the patient can gain a certain clarity as conflict around the theme of mobility, which has existed unconsciously for so long, erupts in the legs, the symbolic location of motion. The vital force, which should flow freely, stops, coagulates, and reveals that, figuratively speaking, many things have gotten stuck, run aground, or been inhibited. The ability to change one's viewpoint and incorporate new views of life may be lost, and one's opinion about life may *coagulate* into a prejudice. The stagnation of the blood indicates how stubborn the patient is about his vital force. He counters Heraklit's words that "everything flows" with his own words "everything stagnates." While Heraklit described the phenomenon of life, the patient exists in a state of nonliving while still being alive. Flowing requires constant transformation and adaptation to ever-changing circumstances. The fact that a person has stopped flowing and stopped changing becomes apparent through an obstructed flow in the body.

The anatomical condition following thrombosis also serves to clarify some issues. The obstruction of a vessel creates a dead-end for the vital force. In this hopeless situation, under the pressure of congestion, the organism attempts to help itself by adopting a "policy of little steps." New vascular connections, called *anastomoses,* are formed, and bridges are built to vessels that are still functioning. In this way, the vital force is brought to its goal via detours and hidden paths. This suggests an avenue for therapy, in the figurative sense, that involves finding new paths for the life energy, and creating new connections that can build bridges within the conscious mind. Another route out of this dead-end involves reorganization of the thrombosis. Small vessels begin to grow through the dam created by the blood clot, forming a vascular network and reinstating the lost connections. Once again, the hypotensive patient with weak connective tissue must accomplish this with small steps and modest solutions.

The most dangerous complication of deep-vein thrombosis is a *pulmonary embolism,* which further reduces communication by shutting down the lungs, the organ of exchange. If exchange is no longer taking place on the emotional level, the body must take extreme measures. In a desperate attempt to call attention to this tragedy, the body sacrifices this exchange.

5.

Therapies for Low Pressure and Connective Tissue

The approach of orthodox medicine to low blood pressure does not differ significantly from that taken by naturopathy. The measurement of blood pressure is a primary component of diagnosis. If the patient has normal blood pressure despite his complaints, the examination itself may be the cause of his problem through its agitating effect. In this case, he has normal blood pressure because he is facing his problem and, in addition, is facing the doctor (with his problem). With such patients, the so-called "standing test" can be of further assistance. For ten minutes, the patient must stand without support. The typical hypotensive patient will not be able to do so without a loss in blood pressure, thereby revealing his problem as well as his attitude toward life.

With respect to therapy, it is no surprise that the miracle drug is motion. According to current understanding, both orthodox medicine and naturopathy make the same recommendation: physical movement. Once again, this involves an obvious step to the opposite pole, and is only attempted on the physical level. Experience supports this therapy. As long as the patient engages in physical motion, he has no symptoms. However, once he has terminated motion therapy, his symptoms return. Consequently, a gradual increase in training is recommended, which must be maintained on an adequate level for the rest of his life. Starting with walking, the training continues with jogging, swimming, and hiking. Since it is important for the patient to remain in motion for a long period of time, interval training and bodybuilding are less suitable. The smallest interruption of the training program, such as a flu, immediately interrupts the effect, and he must start all over again.

Ultimately, the patient is missing inner emotional movement and mental "strolls," the need for which must first be appreciated. Even though he is not willing to make any effort to train in these areas, the symbolic level can at least be touched through physical exercise. However, these effects do not usually reach much beyond the physical level. Working on the theme in this manner is certainly better than doing nothing, but will not resolve the internal issues. Again, the solution can only be achieved on the inner level.

Even orthodox medical professionals are disappointed with the comfortable path of medication. Klepzig admitted that such remedies have an effect for only about one hour. In addition, the body gets used to these chemicals and becomes increasingly adept at counteracting their effects. It is almost as if the body does not want to let itself be supported in such a commonplace manner.

In addition to their rapidly subsiding effect, medications have the disadvantage of making a patient dependent. Since they lack stability and are constantly searching for reliable support, patients are only too eager to clutch at such straws. Even if their pills no longer have any medicinal effect, these medications have become emotional crutches in the truest sense of the word, and patients can no longer do without them. In this situation, it is only too easy to abuse other "energy-boosters" as well. Coffee, tea, and champagne become crutches that may help patients stand up and walk, but obstruct their independence and long-term progress. Nicotine is a particularly dangerous drug because its effect as an energy-booster is based on illusion; in fact, it worsens the already poor circulation more than does any other drug. The hands and feet get even colder, and communication problems become more apparent.

The medical profession's suggestions regarding therapy for weakness of the connective tissues can be interpreted just as easily. If the tissues can no longer hold and support the expanded, sluggishly meandering veins, supportive stockings or firmly wrapped bandages are used. The inner support is replaced by external means. In this case, too, orthodox medicine admits that chemical medications do not work effectively. Naturopathy has long known about the effects of horse-chestnut extract. The strength and vitality of this would certainly help to solve the problem, but it is not sufficient to apply it externally as an ointment or to swallow it as capsules.

Both medical perspectives are willing to be content with these unsatisfactory results because the entire complex of symptoms is not life-threatening. In fact, hypotension actually increases life expectancy, at least in the quantitative sense. However, qualitatively, patients have little to gain from their sleepy lives. Since quantity ranks higher than quality in modern medicine, and in our modem life style in general, the patients' complaints are not taken seriously, or at least not as seriously as complaints about high blood pressure.

In this point, at least, the patient's expectation is not fulfilled. He would prefer others, and doctors in particular, to pull his chestnuts out of the fire for him. He wants others to do something for him, and to help him move forward, because he is too weak to do so himself. In this respect, orthodox medicine will disappoint him, which is its only true service to this clinical syndrome. Ideally, the mistaken notion that some kind of external solution exists would be dispelled. In the worst case, patients are consoled throughout life by references to their sluggish constitution and are given other "stabilizing" information. However, such stabilization only stabilizes their instability, thus prolonging their time out on the sidelines of animated life.

It is harder, yet more healing, to reject all projections. "Help yourself, or nobody will help you" would be a fitting motto in this case. Neither strenuous research efforts, the doctor's willingness to help, nor a spouse or partner's attempts to play an active role and climb the career ladder will help the hypotensive patient with weak connective tissue to stand on his own two feet. Instead of projecting onto others or escaping to the lively opposite pole, a reconciliation with one's own misery is recommended. The learning task lies in recognizing the symbolism of the illness, and accepting it as a chance to take a first step in the right direction, toward finding one's own direction. Each symptom provides an image that not only reflects the unresolved level that causes suffering, but also provides a resolution that promises redemption from the symptom.

The patient with low blood pressure is virtually forced to the floor. He is beaten down and powerless, if not unconscious. Although this state is humiliating, it offers the opportunity to learn true humility. Acceptance of one's apparent weakness can be the first step in this direction. When the surrounding world is experienced as overpowering, the patient feels small and incapable. Yet, realizing one's own smallness in comparison with the wonders of Creation, and accepting it, is the precondition for humbleness. This humility requires a step hypotensive patients are close to taking; the step away from bravery, arrogance, and boldness and toward humility. While courage involves the will to fight and rebel within, the pupil of humility must learn to submit himself, and to consciously give in without resentment. The hypotensive patient is already so close to this state that he only needs to consciously accept what is already constantly happening to him. He needs to consciously stand up for what he is already doing most of the time, which is lying at the feet of the world, humbling himself before everyone and everything.

Saints such as Saint Francis of Assisi and Saint Claire made such exercises part of their spiritual path. In this way, they found *fulfillment* instead of *overfilling* their veins. Like a snail, the retreat into one's own center has to be accepted, and one's life must be lived out consciously, taking care of everything at a snail's pace, yet steadily, like the totem animal. The hermitage inside one's house should be put to use, and ultimately even enjoyed. In the long run, the greatest opportunities for development lie within oneself, rather than in the external world. If everything constantly turns black before the external eyes, this can be seen as a challenge to learn to look with the inner eyes and to let oneself be cushioned and carried by Mother Earth. Dizzy spells are a test for the conscious letting go of power and of all demands on the symbolic physical stage. In this way, the depths of another dimension can be reached.

This recommendation may sound extreme in an age that sets its stakes on the power of the feasible. On the other hand, it is no more radical than the life patients are forced to live because of their symptoms. Voluntarily accepting what has forced itself on oneself, and cannot be changed anyhow, requires no religious conviction but simply healthy common sense. All the symptoms point in this one direction.

Although an uneventful life may be frustrating, it is the starting point for many seekers to embark on a richer and more colorful inner life. Constantly having heavy feet that are tired of walking drags a person down, in his mood as well as in the concrete sense. At the same time, however, it brings one closer to Mother Earth, the feminine pole and source of all life. When these "lead feet" are experienced consciously, a feeling of being rooted and connected with the earth can develop. This is suggested both by the earth's gravity and by the corresponding heaviness of the feminine water element, which has become congested in the legs. Mother Earth, so to speak, calls her children back to her. Even the loops of the meandering veins draw archetypal feminine patterns that contrast with masculine straightness. Dizziness exemplifies the same circular motion, only on a less concrete level. Consciously letting oneself be spun around and finding one's place in the *circle* of natural life may be the hidden learning task. By permitting such feminine symbolic power to have an effect on the emotional level would provide relief at the physical level.

On the emotional level, physical delicacy and impressionability can be recognized as sensitivity and sensitiveness. Softness and a lack of boundaries can become adaptability, elasticity, and flexibility. The refusal to fight against physical limitations can lead to the conscious renunciation of emotional boundaries and, furthermore, to limitless love. Misery can grow into *misericordia*, that is compassion, and the perception that all life involves suffering can lead to the realization that all life deserves compassion. Thus, the misery of hypotension leads the patient to one of Buddha's fundamental teachings.

The demands of these learning tasks illustrate how much one can achieve if one consciously takes them on. A person who concentrates on the center of his snail's house, and creates order within it, will ultimately discover his own heart. The archetypal pattern of the spiral guarantees this. Everything else will evolve automatically out of this center, even all the desired qualities of the opposite pole, such as the ability to act, steadfastness, mobility, and magnanimity. Any courage that evolves from true humility is essentially different from the brashness with which the hypertensive patient wants to lift the world out of its hinges. If a person penetrates his weaknesses and surrenders to them, he will find that unequaled strength lies beyond.

An Eastern metaphor clarifies this. The Tai-Chi master is so yielding in his movements, so flowing and supple, that the little bird who has perched on his shoulder can no longer fly away. Every time it wants to push off, the master's shoulder gives way. The bird is captured and deprived of its power by this very softness. The power of violence and battle could not have achieved what is no more than child's play for the power of total surrender.

This timeless wisdom takes form in the Tai-Chi symbol (Illustration 5). Within the deepest feminine yin one finds the opposite pole of masculine yang, and vice versa. If the feminine turns itself completely inward and becomes increasingly feminine, it must ultimately encounter strength at its core. This strength will

Heart-Aches

not be in the form of boasting or strong-arming, but the true inner power. This knowledge is the basis of the Christian instruction: "If any one strikes you on the right cheek, turn to him the other also." Whoever is capable of living from his innermost feeling is further along on the path and more powerful than one who is only apparently powerful and immediately hits back with physical strength.

Both sociological factors and the distribution of hypotension make its learning tasks more difficult. Low blood pressure is a symptom that predominates among women, while the opposite pole, high blood pressure, is found more frequently among men. All the primary learning tasks that result from the symptoms of hypotension sound like a mockery of feminist objectives and this movement's goal of emancipation. Feminists want to get out of the snail's house, remove this form of dependency, and act freely and independently. Their ideal is a male one, and they attempt to acquire male-dominated positions of power. With low blood pressure, however, this is a hopeless venture; the woman is caught by her constitution and must outrun her own shadow. Although this desire is a courageous dream, one's shadow cannot be outrun. At best, it can be redeemed—which is difficult enough.

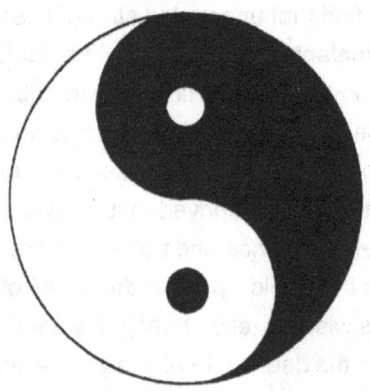

Illustration 5

These comments are not intended as a judgment of the feminist movement, except perhaps to say that its goals are understandably, as are all yearnings for the opposite pole. Its goals, however, require women with weak circulation to take a second step before the first one has been accomplished. If one's physical inheritance includes a soft, feminine charisma, with blond hair, blue eyes, freckles, weak connective tissue, and a tendency toward low blood pressure, the learning task is to live out this kind of femininity and redeem it. The desired power will ultimately evolve from the center of femininity, rather than by attending seminars on rhetoric or bodybuilding classes.

Of course, every woman also has a masculine pole, called the animus by C.G. Jung, Just as every man has a feminine part, called the anima. Generally, the first task is to live out and redeem the part presented through one's own gender, especially if this part is strongly emphasized by one's physical characteristics. However, the symptoms themselves provide the most definitive guideposts, because they indicate what portion of the life task has been suppressed in the shadow and is now pleading for deliverance.

6.

Hypertension—Life Under Pressure

6.1 Figures and Symptoms

A patient is diagnosed with high blood pressure if his blood pressure readings consistently exceed 140/90 mm Hg. Today, eighty million Americans suffer from high blood pressure, numbers that illustrate the extent of this symptom. Woeful terms for hypertension range from "public enemy number one" to the "epidemic of the century." No other symptom takes so many lives and costs so much money. Patients with high blood pressure have heart attacks three times more frequently, and strokes four times more frequently, than do others. The money spent on this disease and the resulting lost income are astronomical. Thus, this illness fulfills all the prerequisites of a scourge in modern industrial society.

Its causes, however, are so closely associated with the living conditions of our society that the medical profession has not been able to clearly distinguish them. Nine out of ten hypertensive patients are diagnosed with so-called *essential hypertension,* which means that no physical cause is known. In plain terms, the diagnosis reveals that medical science does not know what is happening, but prefers to veil this in polite language. The key lies in the term *essential.* In fact, this symptom is essential, meaning vital, for the patient, because it illustrates the essence of his attitude to life.

The difference between the counterpales, hypertension and hypotension, is evident. While low blood pressure produces many dramatic symptoms but is ultimately harmless, high blood pressure hardly shows any symptoms even though it is extremely dangerous.

Compared with a garden hose, the hypotensive patient's circulation corresponds to a wide, limp hose with a fully open nozzle. The water flows out without pressure and, rather than spraying far, falls weakly to the ground right at the nozzle. However, the hypertensive hose is narrow along its entire length, just like the nozzle, and a sharp, thin Jet shoots out. It travels far, but hardly provides any life-giving water. Most of the garden—or body—that is supplied by a hypotensive hose will perish of thirst, since only the zone right at the nozzle receives sufficient water. The garden supplied by a hypertensive hose will also suffer from lack of water, although the little amount that it does provide will be distributed up to the outer boundary. In the center, the heart, the deprivation is most dramatic. Both conditions, therefore, deal with the same problem, even if they are created by opposing characteristics.

To be able to increase blood pressure is essential in life. In situations of extreme demand, it normally increases greatly. In the face of danger, not only do the nerves become tense to a breaking point, but the vessels do so as well. In this case, blood pressure increases to such a degree that the person is literally under pressure. Whether the danger is overcome through flight or attack, the inner pressure decreases to normal values in accordance with the external pressure. When increased secretions of the stress hormone adrenaline are used up, and the blood has fulfilled its task of helping the physical action of the muscles, the organism switches from sympathicotonic tension to vagotonic relaxation.

If this switch to relaxation does not occur, one can assume that the danger has not yet been surmounted, and the conflict remains unresolved. The hypertensive patient lives in this type of situation. His permanent state of sympathicotone tension indicates that he is constantly prepared to fight, or is on the verge of a conflict without ever being able to resolve it. While the hypotensive patient does not confront the matter at hand and immediately runs away, the hypertensive patient is permanently standing next to it. Gun at his side, he expects the attack to take place any minute. Neither person, however, solves the problem through his behavior.

The few symptoms that accompany high blood pressure are related to unexpressed aggression and repressed hostility. Intensified heart palpitations at rest or during minor exertion reveal the sensitive nature of the hypertensive patient. If one's heart is in one's mouth, any expectations are based on fear. Strong heart beats signal intense agitation prior to facing an uncontrollable situation; for example, prior to a test during which the person feels at the mercy of a higher authority. In such situations, many of the hypertensive patient's fears come together at the same time. Namely, he always tries to control and get a grip on things as much possible. The constricted vessels, practically vibrating under controlled tension, reflect this attitude, as does his extreme eagerness to perform. The image of the garden hose with its precise, sharp jet illustrates this situation.

On the other hand, the typical hypertensive patient tends to have problems with authority. Medical studies have established that being at the mercy of an authority one does not accept increases blood pressure. Such a situation "makes one's blood boil" and the less the person admits this to himself, the more his blood pressure will boil. Blood pressure readings for African Americans are on average higher than those for white Americans. African Americans with less education experience hypertension seven times more frequently than do whites with more education. By comparison, blacks in their traditional life-style and surroundings in Africa do not encounter high blood pressure, although authority figures, such as chieftains, are present in that environment as well. However, problems probably do not arise because these authorities are accepted. School dropouts, who often exist in "underdog" situations, tend to have high blood pressure values. Pressure is also highest at the bottom of a pecking order, because it cannot be passed down any further. The symbol of the social pyramid illustrates this fact. Those at the bottom carry everything on their shoulders and, thus, are the most *oppressed*. It is reasonable to assume that hypertensive patients experience life as a continual test, a situation that requires the highest degree of tension and constant readiness to defend oneself.

Hypertensive patients often complain about palpitations during the night, indicating that the vagus does not take control over the combat-ready sympathetic nervous system even at night, the classical time for regeneration. Corresponding dream themes precede the palpitation attacks.

Diminished productivity is usually a relatively late sign of hypertension and can be explained in terms of circulatory problems. As in the example of the garden hose, everything is geared toward high performance but the outcome is only marginal. Even impotence may result. The impotent hypertensive acts as if he is confronting himself, although he actually is not, at least not in the right place. As in hypotension, head pressure may be experienced, indicating where the problem is located, where decisions should be made, and where the problem must be solved. The headache reveals that the patient's basic attitude toward life, which is established in the head, is wrong. Only if an appropriate attitude can be developed will the corresponding position in life be achieved. No matter how much pressure is applied in the wrong place, the patient will not have a breakthrough. Oppressive headaches are often the consequence of too much worry. When someone worries too much, his thoughts revolve around the problem but are unable to solve it. Such is the hypertensive patient's condition.

Nervousness and other signs of overwrought nerves reflect the patient's state of tension. In general, problems should never be pushed to the breaking point, unless one is willing to risk that they will break at some point. The hypertensive patient takes this risk. However, before he is overtaken by a breaking heart, a heart attack, or the bursting blood vessel of a stroke, he experiences a series of warning signals. Symptoms include nerves that are tense to the breaking point, irritability, fits of rage, and lack of concentration, as well as symptoms of the autonomic nervous system. Profuse sweating, for example, reveals the fear that rules his life. Someone who "sweats blood" suffers from panic-stricken fear, but even a cold sweat speaks loud and clear.

Fear is even more evident when observing the narrow vessels. The same condition exists as in the case of a narrow heart and its symptoms of angina pectoris and heart attack. For high blood pressure, this condition extends to the entire body. Narrow vessels always show fear constricting the flow of life. Over the long term, this constriction leads to arteriosclerosis. In the body's upper region, coronary sclerosis can cause calcification of the nervous system's switching center, the brain, while in the lower region, it can cause the leg vessels to petrify through *intermittent claudication*. The first case demonstrates that the patient is no longer progressing in his thoughts; obstruction of any type of progress is evident in the second case. Translated, intermittent claudication means "intermediate limping." The patient can only walk for a short distance before he must take a break until the obstructed blood supply has caught up. No quick movement forward is possible, and any form of climbing is difficult. Even climbing a few steps can strain such as patient's narrow boundaries.

At this stage, the fundamental problem is finally clear: no progress is being made in life. If the person feels he can afford to overlook this situation, he must suffer physically. Failing legs illustrate this, as does the inadequately supplied brain. When the memory grows weak, the most important information is lost, while insignificant, old stories are perfectly retained and told over and over, like a broken record. The hypertensive patient who has the courage to be honest with himself can recognize that he is constantly revolving around his theme, as if hypnotized, without actually tackling it. He is practically bubbling with activity, but missing all the essential points. Lacking the courage to make a decisive attack, he indulges instead in peripheral diligence in order to *suppress* any accusations that he is avoiding the central issue.

One of the few symptoms that is easily distinguished is "red hypertension." These patients, who are usually overweight, signal their importance with extremely red faces. Like the glowing bulb of a lighthouse or red lantern, they demand attention by being both warning and alluring at the same time. Something is always happening around such people, which can be dangerous because of all the activity. Although these people are hardly ruffians, they tend to be filled with hot-air or act like pompous fools. Sometimes, no longer able to hold themselves back, they strike out, at least in the figurative sense. In the worst case, they can do a lot of unnecessary damage. Despite all the pressure, the situation seldom gets vicious, however, because the elephant raging in the china shop is basically good-natured and depends on the attention paid him by the spectators. Ultimately, he fears losing their affection. A person who is full of hot air must let off steam. The greatest damage is generally done to the steamroller himself. If not stopped in time, he will pound away endlessly, until he reaches the grave. This is a high-pressure performance, one that is in search of merit and recognition. The typical red hypertension patient must earn everything by himself, likes to be involved in everything, and considers himself irreplaceable. If a taxi driver were to ask him where he wanted to go, his response would be, "It doesn't matter. Pm needed everywhere!"

The tense circulation of such people is often empathized by conspicuously serpentine temporal arteries. Pulsating temples also heighten the impression of a person who is pulsating and involved with every fiber of his tense heart. What he is involved in is less significant than the fact that it is important. That it is, in essence, a diversion is not so easily recognized. The hypertensive patient generally believes in his self-elected mission and its eminent significance. He fails to recognize the escapism inherent in his furious activity and dogged efforts. If he were to see through them, he would not continue in the same style and speed. Such recognition would be the first step toward improvement.

Fortunately, the red hypertensive patient has a way to let go of some of his excess pressure that does not involve much conscious reflection. He can explode like a pressure cooker. He frequently blows his top, which is much healthier than vessels bursting in, for example, the brain. What he is really capable of can be perceived through these fits of rage, which resemble volcanic eruptions. When he fumes and foams and flings his fury at his surroundings, the boiling aggression within him cannot be overlooked. Just as a pressure cooker is less dangerous after some steam has been let off, the hypertensive patient is more relaxed after his fit. But since he avoids exploding at the appropriate places, the pressure usually builds up quickly afterward. The red bulb gives its warning with good reason: danger of explosion, at any time!

Socially, such fits of rage are not beneficial and can damage the good impression made by his diligent activity and super-human efforts. For this reason, and because his eruptions nearly always strike the wrong people, the hypertensive patient will attempt to close these outlets and hold back. He will only achieve recognition if he attempts to master his temper. After an explosion, he is even more pinched and dogged, and his circulatory problem is more hopeless because it has become even more constricted. Although the surrounding world may find it more pleasant if his congested aggression and inhibited hostility are expressed quietly in his facial features or by grinding his teeth, this is more dangerous for the patient. The pressure cooker that closes all its outlets can no longer hiss and whistle so loudly, but the situation inside is more constricted and unpleasant. The walls must be strengthened to withstand the growing tension. Strengthening of the body's vessels is called arteriosclerosis.

If a person, during the course of his lifetime, masters the flow of vital energy in these areas, he faces a pale future due to increasingly high blood pressure and the calcification of his vessels. Medical science speaks of "pale hypertension" and

Hypertension—Life Under Pressure

sometimes also of "malignant hypertension." Since such patients have almost super-human control, they are well-integrated into a society that places great value on control. They pull themselves together to such an extent that very little life remains. The phenomenon of inner loneliness coupled with well-functioning "social" relationships is evident in these cases. A song by Simon and Garfunkel illustrates this condition: "1 am a rock—I am an island..."

Both red and pale hypertensives are similarly hopeless. While the red hypertensive may burst at any moment, which can be fatal on the level of the vessels, the perspective of the pale hypertensive is one of deadness. Even such drastic prospects are usually not enough to radically change the course of life. Doctors who take their patients seriously, and call a spade a spade, experience time and again that only the heart's cry for help in the form of a heart attack can cause a turn toward consciousness. The patient tends to view all prior warnings as mere challenges. Just like his blood, he is accustomed to running up against resistance and mistakenly hopes he will win at some point. Since he fights everywhere except at the decisive fortress, however, victory is impossible at this level.

6.2 External and Internal Pressure

The most important symptom of the hypertensive patient is pressure. Although the patient himself may not feel it for a long time, others perceive it all the more in his behavior. The vital force is under pressure and with it all the themes related to vitality, although the patient never admits this to himself. Only others, who experience the force in his actions, often feel *oppressed* by the hypertensive patient. Just as the blood stream accepts the resistance of the vessel wall and presses against it, the patient presses against outer resistance and seeks opponents with whom to express his struggle in life. Since he has long been fighting with his back to the wall—and has built walls all around himself—he does not realize his condition. His vascular system is like a cage, and his vital force is trapped in a self- made prison. Studies of hypertensive patients' emotional conditions reveal that they tend to feel like prisoners in their own homes. The parental home, family, and even company where they are employed, are experienced as cages; life consists of moving from one cage to another. Although the patient may find these external prisons oppressive, he fails to consciously confront his fundamental deprivation of liberty. Ultimately, this theme sinks into his body. The narrower the prison walls become, the higher the pressure. This law of physics has a direct effect on the rate at which calcification of the walls progresses and elasticity is lost.

This principle applies in the social arena as well. When people are crammed tightly together in places such as prisons, blood pressure rises and leads to increased aggression. Lynch states that blood pressure reflects the harmony between a person and the world beyond his social membrane. Abnormally high pressure on the vessel wall corresponds to pressure in the social environment. Pathophysiological studies show that high blood pressure can even damage the uppermost layer of the vessel wall- the intima. Similarly, high social pressure can damage the structure of relationships when people are crammed in a small space. This could be a reason for the increasing trend toward high blood pressure. More and more people are being brought together in dense centers of population. They work in open-plan offices and recover from work in huge residential complexes. Their apartments, like concrete .shoe boxes, separate them from each other while keeping them contained in the smallest possible space. Such a policy of "apartheid" is the only way to keep so many people together in such a small space. The parallel with domestic animals, such as pigs and cows, is alarmingly clear. Cardiovascular problems are increasing among these animals as well, and more than a few modern pigs die of heart attacks. So that they can bear the stress, psychopharmaceutical drugs are increasingly prescribed for these animals, just as for humans. No wonder things accumulate and calcify in the relationships and vessels of people who are kept in such congested conditions.

Since abnormal pressure in the circulation also puts pressure on the heart and inner center, it is not surprising that the themes of the heart include oppression. Although an intense, inner pressure to produce results may, at times, help one progress in work, it is virtually lethal for the theme of love. This starts at the physical level, the level of sexuality, where a certain physical pressure is necessary but emotional tension prevents the enjoyment of sex. As already mentioned, this can gradually develop into impotence. On the emotional level, this problem gets worse because one cannot function well under pressure. If oppression and tightness replace love and expansiveness, the hypertensive patient will feel depressed and deeply empty, despite his outer activities and importance. The deeper meaning of life is literally crushed and flattened. In order to know the depression of the hypertensive patient, one must come close to him, which is difficult. On the outside, he will keep smiling as long as possible. However, this outer friendly show corresponds to inner *oppression,* and often to a well-restrained hostility against himself and others. In this way, the hypertensive patient creates a double-bind situation: he feels the opposite of what he permits others to see and hear. Children and sensitive adults do not know how to react to him because, no matter what they do, it is always wrong. Animals and less sensitive adults have an easier lime. Animals react to the honest emotional message, while adults respond to the dishonest verbal information.

Even if the hypertensive patient's behavior appears powerful or extreme, a tense and exhausted person is concealed behind it. True relaxation is impossible, although it usually comes into play later, in its most modest form, as depression. This occurs when the emptiness behind the patient's steamroller politics becomes clear as a result of some, usually external, circumstance. A midlife crisis often provides such a circumstance, revealing the full pressure of work, performance, and competition—as well as forceful effort and *expressed* ambition—in a new, less radiant light. Blood pressure often gets out of control precisely at the moment a patient has gotten all external matters under control. In retrospect, life appears as a chain of confined situations in which he had to constantly pull himself together or hold onto himself, while at the same time he could hardly hold himself back or keep his feelings in check. Furthermore, all this was only for the purpose of pressing someone else against the wall—a wall that he had against his own back all along. It also becomes clear that all the pressure he exercised on himself and on the environment ultimately prevented the expression of those things that concerned his heart. Suddenly, he must admit that everything that was impressive, forceful, and emphatic was only a means of evasion.

Such perceptions are oppressive and can even be shattering. However, reconciliation with one's own pattern can result from such despondency. A depressive mood is an honest starting point for a path out of the continual crisis. Besides, the despondent mood has dominated from beneath the surface all along. Even if one could hide this mood from oneself, it would be conspicuous to those who are close.

6.3 Hypertension and Communication—The Language of the Heart

The emotional condition of the hypertensive patient has been explained in the chapter on *The Narrow Heart*. It corresponds to the type A person described there. Some of the most prominent characteristics of hypertensive patients are discussed in detail here.

Perhaps the most peculiar symptom of these patients is their style of communication. Lynch[19] who has published many studies and an entire book on this topic, states: "Finally, we understood that the human circulatory system achieves much more than just adapting to inner and outer requirements: *it also communicates.* Since our hearts speak a language which no one hears or sees and consequently nobody understands, we suffer from heart disease." In his work as professor of psychophysiology, Lynch realized that nothing increases blood pressure as much as speaking. Speech is always connected to the expiratory stream. In terms of physics, it is based on exerting pressure to the outside. In contrast, listening is a passive act of opening and letting in. In symbolic terms, speaking is closer to the Martian principle of attack, while listening is closer to the Venusian principle of love.

Speaking is the most uniquely human form of communication and begins at a very young age. The citing of an infant is part of this as well; Lynch discovered that this form of communication can increase blood pressure. Communication is absolutely vital to life, as proven by the famous historical experiment in which a king wished to find the original language of humanity. He arranged for a group of children to receive attention in every possible way by absolutely speechless servants. But, instead of revealing the original language, the children died. Experience with children in foster homes today reveals the importance of communication in general, as well as the specific role of loving communication for the health of children.

After birth, the close physical connection between mother and child through the umbilical cord is replaced by an emotional bond. The importance of this for the growth of the human being is demonstrated by all the unfortunate children whose bond was destroyed. Later in life, the first bond is replaced by a social bond with others. This is also vital for life, as shown by experiences in solitary isolation. Such isolation can be torture. Conversation is the lifeline that connects adults with each other.

The crying of a baby is a plea for affection. Something is de-*pressing* the baby, who starts crying in order to *express* this situation. At the same time, rapidly rising blood pressure reflects this oppression on the physical level. When a person screams later in life, the situation is similar. She feels oppressed in some way and expresses this in her scream. She wishes to gain attention and, as a result, relaxation of her tension.

The results of Lynch's research can be interpreted to mean that, because speaking gradually takes over the role of crying, the crying indicated oppression in the first place. Crying can be understood as an attempt to gain relief, to let off steam, and to express oneself. Above all, the fact that blood pressure rises relatively independently of the contents of the speech supports this assumption. In the history of evolution, content was added at a relatively late point in time. Long before the child speaks in a way that can be understood intellectually, she talks in a language that is without recognizable content to adults. She expresses something without concrete meaning. In the course of adult life, because of the increasing importance of intellectual messages, she gradually forgets the emotional character of language as an outlet for oppression and as an emotional bond with others. The more this emotional aspect of language recedes into the background, the less a person can express herself completely. This increases her chances of keeping the pressure to herself and renouncing any form of relief.

Keeping this in mind, it is also understandable that Lynch found the highest increase in blood pressure during telephone calls. Since phoning is essentially an act of conveying information, the emotional contact, as well as the aspect of body language and nonverbal expression, is pushed into the background. In comparison, "conversations" with small children can create emotional relief because the emotional aspects are in the foreground. Furthermore, authority problems are not triggered for an adult who is speaking to children. In this respect, even pets have an influence that reduces blood pressure, according to Lynch. If a person can speak lovingly to another living being who is "lower" than himself, he can reduce his blood pressure. On the other hand, if he speaks "up" to someone, which generally connotes a higher authority, his blood pressure rises.

In this context, the hypertensive patient's style of speaking is impressive because it differs from a normal speaking style. In general, when a person opens his mouth during a conversation, he intends to immediately make himself and the matter at hand understood by the listener. Even the first few words are an invitation to enter his world of thoughts and images. In the case of the hypertensive person, this is not so. As soon as he begins to speak, something within him chokes up—namely, his vessels. He uses words that keep the person he is talking to at a distance. Rattling on and on, his words bubble out with breathless, controlled urgency and spill onto his surroundings like a torrent.

Hypertensive patients often speak without pausing, without even stopping to breathe. Therefore, it is almost impossible to interrupt them; they must be cut short. It is very difficult to match them in a confrontation with words. Since they do not permit the other person to speak, it is difficult to finish one's sentences in a conversation with them. Words become weapons with which they attack and walls behind which they hide. Their reactions come like *shots*. Conversations are the main battleground for many hypertensive patients, and the art of contradicting is one of their favorite activities, in accordance with their theme that "the best should also know everything." If their arguments are met with strong opposing force, they increase the speed and intensity of their speech in order to put more pressure behind their words.

While he can talk well, the hypertensive patient is a poor listener. Because of his negative expectations, he attempts to catch any signs of the speaker's possible antagonism early enough that he can be better armed for a counter blow. In this attempt to immediately detect any attack, he often reads one into the other person's words. The result is a degenerating form of communication that does not allow the deeper feelings that resonate with words to be heard. This can no longer be called a dialog (the Greek *did* means "through") because the messages no longer penetrate the hypertensive patient's protective armor. For a true dialog, the counterpole is necessary: openness.

Considering the opposite pole further clarifies this interpretation. In heart-to-heart communication, feelings are reflected in the words that are taken to heart. This type of communication seeks harmony instead of war. Its objective is to convey something, instead of creating confrontation; cooperation takes the place of battle. In such a conversation, listening is as important as talking. Two people share a common topic. The hypertensive patient, however, primarily puts out words and hardly listens. If his opponent succeeds in taking the floor, he is already considering how to counter.

During phases of relaxed listening in normal conversation, blood pressure falls to its resting level. One can use pauses that occur naturally while breathing to relax. If such moments are missing, considerable pressure builds up; for example, in the case of the hypertensive patient who avoids pausing for breath or who does not relax while listening, but defensively awaits his next opportunity to speak. Lynch has proven convincingly how dangerous such conversations are for patients with high blood pressure. The pressure, which is already at a high level, rises far more rapidly and intensely than for people with sound circulatory systems. A typical sign is exhaustion after the conversation. At this point, the deep wisdom "silence is golden" is easily understood.

Meditating on this familiar maxim can give wings to the constricted, depressed soul of the hypertensive patient. It is almost impossible to draw conclusions about his inner feeling by merely observing the expression on his face or his gestures. He prefers to show a "poker face" and does not even notice if all hell has broken loose in his vessels. Lynch designed a psychotherapy for such people in which they monitor their blood pressure during a conversation. When their blood pressure peaks, they can use simple breathing exercises to immediately calm it down. Over many hours, they learn to keep their blood pressure in check, thus permitting greater freedom and relaxation.

When two such high-pressured talkers meet, things usually happen fast. A vehement exchange of blows is one possible result, although not the most likely. Cynical barbs and words that obscure more than they reveal are another specialty among such people. Often, these partners in conversation are fooled without their even noticing it, at least not in time. Politicians and managers are good subjects to study if one wants to understand this type of one-sided, snappy conversation.

The separation of emotions from language is a problem shared by many psychosomatically ill people. This is especially evident in people suffering from hypertension, who are generally unaware of their own feelings. Before they can regain their split off emotions, they need to take an inventory of the status quo and reconcile themselves with it. They must become conscious of their overexertion. Observing this, psychoanalyst Condrau[20] commented: "In essence, a person is only overexerted if he resists what is occupying him, or if he is so completely absorbed by these demands that he becomes a slave to them and any further free development is impossible." Hypertensive patients can be affected by both variations. Their resistance to the stream of life is evident in their resisting vessels as well as in the resistant manner with which they carry on a conversation. They let themselves become so absorbed by the demands they feel that everything else pales in comparison. Even their closest family relationships and the most central aspects of life, such as matters of the heart, are unimportant to hypertensive patients who try to ramrod their goals with excessive pressure.

The high degree of suppressed aggression and self-control that Franz Alexander,[21] a pioneer in psychosomatic medicine, referred to in his studies should be recognized in this context as well. This form of suppression is easier to achieve in red hypertension than in pale hypertension. In the former, barbs, cynical statements, and other forms of aggression must be taken into account. The deeply oppressive loneliness created by these self-imposed communication barriers must be recognized. Furthermore, hypertension thrives on omnipresent competitive pressure and the ambition to always be number one. The one who is first is consequently always alone. The closed boundaries that constrict the self must also be inspected and accepted, starting with the vascular system. The emotional and social boundaries must be discovered as well.

Ultimately, a desire for recognition underlies all this tension and overexertion. The motto that "love must be earned" does not permit love to just happen. Although this motto implies that love is in the number one position, it actually obstructs love. We have described love as unconditional openness and expansiveness. However, the hypertensive patient attempts to fight for love by narrow means and by closing himself off. He places his stake in the battle on Mars, the God of War and the natural antagonist of Venus, the Goddess of Love. The hypertensive patient makes the classic mistake of expecting recognition and love from the outside, thus overlooking that love can only come within. Actively opening oneself and expanding, opens the gate for love to enter. On the other hand, tension and exertion narrow and close a person, thereby chasing away the Goddess of Love. This combination of desire for love and aggressive ambition are evident in typical hypertensive phrases such as: "I'm married to my job."

Finally, the site of these events is also worth a closer look. The circulatory system, which is responsible for connection and exchange within the body, indicates through its constriction and, later hardening, where the problem lies. The flow of communication is obstructed and artificially choked; in the worst case, it is strangled. However, the simple language of the organs makes translation into the figurative level easy. While the hypotensive patient is obstructed in communication due to his lack of effort, the hypertensive patient blocks communication through overexertion. The heart is endangered by both these communication barriers because both carry the threat of a heart attack. Again, for most hypertensive patients, the decisive area is their inner center, which they do not face despite all the trouble. In order to divert attention away from their center and all its uncontrollable emotions, they spare no efforts, even if it means leading an unbelievably exerting and depressing life.

6.4 The Redemption of Pressure—A Chance for Development

Once one has perceived the basic pattern and, no matter how difficult it may be, has recognized it as one's own, one can also successfully work through the pressing themes on the more resolved levels. The resolved forms of fear and constriction have already been outlined in the chapter *The Narrow Heart* as concentration and wise, essential limitation. For hypertensive patients, the circulation and the communication system with its center, the heart, are most essential.

For red hypertension, rising anger is often the force that can induce a reversal. This form of anger is not negative, but rather a vast, wrongly directed form of potential energy. Instead of suppressing it, which only raises blood pressure, it can be redirected and ignited in the right way. For example, instead of blowing up at a member of one's family who is not responsible for the problem, it is more appropriate to attack the source of the anger, perhaps one's boss at work or a member of the family who is responsible. This requires courage and, in some circumstances, a willingness to look for a more suitable job afterward.

Regarding weight, only the levels need to be changed. Everyone wants to be important, but it must be clear whether physical expression is enough or another form of '"weight" is preferred. Perhaps there are more important themes than eating or expanding of one's physical sphere of influence.

A red face discloses the rush of blood to the highest area of the body. It is worth considering the level on which this symptom occurs. A red face is Just one way of signaling that a person has brains. But, as is the case for an excited turkey, something besides burning rage or fiery zeal may cause the red face. For example. Just as a turkey puffs itself up when it has sexual expectations, many people also get a fire-red face during such moments. If the conspicuous coloration of the face proves to be a sign of unadmitted, continual courtship—like those red lanterns in front of obvious "rutting places"—it is possible to enjoy the chronic tension of expectation and, thus, transform it into a means of relaxation.

Whatever the central issue, whether an outrageous boss or one's embarrassing erotic needs, it is definitely not a mistake to pay close attention to the theme, which could be decisive for the heart. Heartfelt rage and love both have a liberating and opening effect, which is why they are healthy. However, even extensive activity in other innocuous areas will not create (re)solution.

Problems with authority are directly related. Grumbling about one's boss does no good when he is not present. The hypertensive patient's strength is precisely that he does not release his excessive pressure except when it is not dangerous to do so. However, such explosions are of little use to him. Every explosion provides at least temporary relief, but those of greatest value can be both dangerous and relieving. One's own authority can also be a source of learning. It is helpful for the hypertensive patient to truly bond with another person, instead of having many superficial acquaintances, and to have a single deep love relationship instead of many oppressive relationships. However, this requires him to take a daring step out of the pecking order and become an equal partner. As long as he puts himself above others, they will place themselves above him as well; as long as he pecks, he also will be pecked.

It should be easy to see through the ambition to reach the absolute top. After all, there can only be one such unique position on earth. In statistical terms, the chances of achieving this position are one in over five billion. On the other hand, one should consider, if one has not already done so, whether this position is not already occupied—by God. If a person can recognize the highest authority and be reconciled with it, his annoyance with any small, worldly superiors will melt like butter in the sun. If the highest level still seems too distant, the person will profit from tangling with the next highest authority, whether in the family, school, business, or wherever he is fighting at the time.

Of course, refraining from aggressive behavior saves the lives of countless spouses and superiors every day. However,

Hypertension—Life Under Pressure

one can never completely refrain from aggression. If one does not vent one's anger, it will inevitably escape in small but well-aimed doses through sharp words that are full of barbs, and no less hurtful. Instead of plugging up these outlets by pulling oneself together, it is better to channel one's anger into more important and useful areas. Rather than constantly attack another person's tolerance, for example, one could shoot at the frontiers of science. By applying the *sharpness* of one's mind in this way, one may even earn some credit, thus achieving the recognition one so fervently desires—and maybe even a trace of love as well. Consciousness could also be applied to verbal attacks by using them satirically toward "bad politicians" and other grievances that burn in one's soul. However, it is important to perform this exercise as an end in itself, and not for a "good cause."

One can become conscious of one's aggressions by recognizing the injuries one has caused others. When it becomes clear that these injuries inevitably hit back in one way or another, one will naturally wish to refrain from causing painful verbal injury. Consciously retrieving one's aggression in this way is an enormous step forward from an unconsciously suppressed state of mind. While no longer hurting anyone, the patient is able to work on this theme.

The continuous flow of words, uninterrupted by doubts or breathing, can also promote development if one talks about what is truly essential—namely that which originate in his heart. To learn how to express oneself is distinctly healing. The therapy successes reported by Lynch show that it is appropriate to let off pressure, and thereby reach the relaxed counterpole where feelings color a conversation and one is able to enjoy oneself. Although less pressure is produced, more can be gained in the figurative sense. Even the act of giving time and attention to one's partner in the conversation shows greater openness and contrasts with old patterns of limitation and exclusion.

In addition, Lynch's therapies demonstrate the futility of speaking breathlessly while consciously controlling blood pressure; no one wants to increase his blood pressure in such a suicidal manner. Overemphasizing one pole of reality only reveals the opposite pole. The deeper one breathes in, the more certain it is that an exhalation will follow. Excessively overstepping the mark will certainly result in exhaustion. The attempt to consciously bubble out words without taking a breath in between leads to a conscious pause in breathing. Any form of directing consciousness toward the breathing process can contribute to a reversal of polarity. If one spends his life holding his breath it is, by definition, no life. A simple experiment can clarify this. If one decides afterward to continue living, a consciously deep breath is both an easy and convincing way to do so. In the beginning, one will realize repeatedly in the middle of a conversation that one is attempting to hold one's breath, and thus kill oneself. Simple realization of this fact will set breathing back into motion. Breathing is life. Flat, suppressed breathing represents a flat, suppressed life, while every conscious breath brings depth to life. If one breathes consciously despite problems of high blood pressure, even the realm of spiritual liberation will ultimately be opened. In this respect, the value of simply listening to one's breathing for hours, days, or even weeks at a time—a customary practice of Zazen—becomes clear.

To escape from living in the cage of his own narrow vascular system, the patient has to change levels while working on this principle. If, on the outside, he plays the world conqueror with extensive connections and immeasurable influence, his body is forced to correct the problem in its own way by becoming a narrow, cramped vascular cage. It would be healthier to limit himself on the outside, while creating more freedom and open communication in the vascular system. Fantastic connections to "God and the world" are of little use if it is not to the one God, and if the vessels in the body close up. However, one can live very well even in the tiniest chamber if inner expansiveness is ensured. For example, Sri Aurobindo and other Indian gurus lived for years in one small room without feeling the least bit confined. Such extremes are only meant to illustrate the principle, however; it is not necessary to imitate them.

Going too far in the other direction can also lead to extremes. In this case, the meditation corner is replaced by the hospital room, but the principle remains the same; the person takes no more steps into the outer world and has abundant time to think about inner expansion. This reduction in space can nurture the principle of constriction in an ideal way, especially if it is focused on what is truly essential—one's own heart.

In this sense, the feeling of undergoing a continual test, a fear from which hypertensive patients often suffer, can become productive. From an esoteric religious perspective, life is one big school with an abundance of tests. If one grants the highest test authority to the divine power, proving oneself to the rest of the world is not longer necessary'. Recognizing that one is in God's hands, one will see that no boss or authority figure is omnipotent. Then, even the most excessive demands become acceptable. Submitting oneself to the highest divine authority is always an excessive demand, but a very productive one. One might fail repeatedly, but one will learn from every mistake. With every "disillusion," one will put an end to the big illusion about the nature of this world.

Even the feeling of loneliness can take us a step further in this process because, in addition to its oppressive meaning, it contains the idea of solitude (sole-itude). This represents the opportunity to limit oneself to one thing and to bring this one thing to fruition. Similarly, aloneness (all-one-ness) offers the possibility of being everything in one. According to Lynch's studies, the loneliness patients suffer is the decisive factor in cardiovascular disease. The heart breaks most often when people are unattached or alone. Voluntarily chosen solitude on the spiritual path, however, is an excellent form of protection. Trappist monks who maintained silence for an entire lifetime had no indication of cardiovascular problems. In their *lone*liness, the One stood in the center, and they waked the path to all-one-ness. Instead of standing alone at the center of attention, it is more beneficial for body and soul to place the One at the center of life.

Heart-Aches

This allows the unanswered scream of high blood pressure to be heard. Accepting one's symptoms, and living consciously with respect to the patterns connected with them, can lead to liberation. If the patient enters the battle at the decisive point, the point where she is required to be, she can *express* her inner pressure in a creatively forceful manner. After the heroic battle has been won, relaxation will follow of its own accord. Of course, it is difficult for such a *high-pressure* person to realize that she is avoiding the topic. If she confronts herself, she will eventually find the sleeping dragon waiting to be conquered. In every aspect of conflict—from being tense, to exerting oneself, to relaxation after the battle—one may encounter archetypal human history and find the opportunity to transform hypertensive symptoms into something productive for one's evolutionary path.

7.

High and Low Pressure—Hand in Hand

The hypotensive patient lives in a space that is too wide for him, symbolized by the blood losing its way in the expansiveness of the vascular system. The restricting, supportive element is lacking in his life. He may even develop agoraphobia and feel overwhelmed by expansiveness and open areas. The consequences are despondency, hopelessness, and resignation. In contrast, the hypertensive patient feels imprisoned in a space that is too tight for him. It frightens him and constantly obstructs his development. Like the claustrophobic, he feels restricted, constrained, and limited in expressing himself. On closer examination, one can see that these patients press themselves into a frame that is too small for them and their demands.

Both types of patients share the problem of choosing a space that is appropriate for them. This can be understood by imagining a train compartment. The hypotensive tends to hide away in a corner, hoping the other passengers will leave him alone if he avoids eye contact with them. He would never stretch his legs into the space of the person across from him or extend beyond his place. The hypertensive, on the other hand, tends to occupy a place in the middle where he sits at the center of attention and has everyone else under visual control. He likes to set the tone of the conversation, and it does not bother him if his possessions occupy the neighboring seat as well. However, he would feel constricted if anybody else took such liberties.

Precisely because they are such opposites, both types of patients tend to engage in some similar actions, because ultimately they are connected by the same theme. The hypertensive likes to rip open the window, even if this is somewhat inconsiderate, because he feels too constricted in the little compartment. The hypotensive also likes to open the window because it provides an escape for him and because he is not forced to breathe the same air as the other passengers. For him, solidarity with the others quickly becomes too obligatory. However, he would never act inconsiderately. If he senses even the slightest resistance, he will do without the air, suffering in silent resignation because he feels he is at other people's mercy.

Similarities, such as where and how to sit down, reveal that neither of these two types has found his place in life. In his modesty and insecurity, the hypotensive tends to sit on the edge of the chair, thus signaling that he is not even considering committing himself or taking a position. Instead, he would give way to someone who is stronger (a hypertensive, for example). But the hypertensive also prefers to sit at the edge of his chair. After all, he must always be on the go. Rest and relaxation are not possible for him. Both these types cannot set themselves—and the burden of their body—down, but remain sitting on their problem.

In their contrary natures, both types share some mutual themes. Both get dizzy easily, which reveals their problem with uprightness. Their tendency toward insincerity and a more earthy approach to things provides them both with needed time for reflection. In addition to their problem with uprightness, patients with high and low blood pressure share the problem of finding meaning. While the resigned hypotensive no longer finds meaning in anything, the hypertensive, who is overly tense, no longer sees the meaning of life due to his stubbornness.

High and Low Pressure—Hand in Hand

In accordance with the motto *birds of a feather flock together,* these two types like to get together. Another saying, *opposites attract,* also indicates that they are made for each other because of their contrasting behavior. In this case, the woman is almost always in the hypotensive—and the man in the hypertensive—role, which is not surprising because their symptoms are strongly gender-specific. According to the popular game of "projection," she expects him to live out the dynamics that she is missing, and to climb the social ladder of success, because she cannot even stand up on her own two feet. He is quite enthusiastic about this task because he cannot stand to be confined by domestic life for very long. In his irritable, overwrought slate, her boring sleepiness is soothing. Of course, there are some drops of bitterness in this idyllic relationship. With his tactless sharpness, he often places unreasonable demands on someone who is almost dying from too much sensibility and sensitivity. No wonder she suffers emotionally when her unstable connective tissue is constantly confronted with his bulging fullness that practically bursts at the seams.

It is only natural that a small, weak, pale woman innocently looks for a "real" man to give her the stability she is missing and the strength to master life. The man, for his part, desires to protect her from the rigors of the world. For her, of course, the partner is the opposite pole and, thus, the better half of herself. The only factor that complicates this is that, ultimately, each individual must find everything within and live it out. The partner reflects one's shadow, the parts of the soul that are not lived and often are vehemently rejected. This is why relationships are so important and so difficult at the same time. The opposite pole is the distant goal that one cannot ignore, but which must wait until one has recognized, accepted, and resolved the learning task at hand. Since the gender distribution of these medical problems is so clear, it is evident that women should first develop their feminine aspect, and men should resolve their masculine aspect.

Since society primarily suffers from the masculine pole, which is unresolved and has gone to extremes, one can see how menacing the problem of high blood pressure is and how relatively untroublesome—and, consequently, disturbing but harmless—the unresolved feminine pole remains. This has not always been the case, which suggests a correlation between our high-pressured society and its most dangerous symptom. Hypertension has virtually become the symbol of this society and this era. It is a well-known phenomenon that every culture produces its own typical diseases. Older physicians report that in Germany during the period of economic depression and lethargy directly after World War n, their waiting rooms were full of patients with low blood pressure. With the currency reform and economic recovery, things began to cheer up—for blood pressure as well. This was necessary at the time, and perhaps suggests the question we should ask today: Could we have overdone things a bit and should we not allow things to settle down again—blood pressure and society in general?

8.

Further Problems in the Course of the Circle

In addition to essential hypertension, which makes up the lion's share of all types of hypertension, several other forms of high blood pressure are related to diseases of other organs. Hypertension caused by the kidneys must be mentioned, as well as high blood pressure accompanying coarctation of the aorta. A tumor of the adrenal medulla, a *pheochromocytoma,* can also create hypertension. Other forms of high blood pressure in general can be interpreted in the same way as essential hypertension if they produce the same symptoms. The meaning of the primarily affected organ must be included in the interpretation as well.

Since the circulation connects all the organs, tissue, and cells, it is obvious that it is also involved in all clinical syndromes. Any comprehensive work-up must deal with all possible medical problems. In the case of fever, for example, circulatory reactions are in the foreground. However, fever is primarily connected with inflammation. In comparison, although hemorrhoids are true vascular disorders, they are primarily a problem in relation to digestion. The clinical syndrome of migraine also has its basis in the vascular system, but nevertheless is a form of headache.

Heart-Aches

Even though stroke is a problem of blood flow in purely physiological terms, its effects touch the neurological field. Although the phenomenon of blushing (discussed in the section on red hypertension) is a circulatory symptom, it cannot be considered a circulatory disease.

In contrast, Raynaud's disease is a true circulatory disorder with such symptoms as sudden paleness and numbness of the fingers. There is a smooth transition to this condition from so-called *digiti mortui,* the dead finger. In this case, the individual fingers suddenly turn pale, cold, numb, and stiff due to coldness or "nervous influence." It affects girls and young women almost exclusively. Orthodox medicine recommends warmth, but is otherwise reserved in its recommendations due to the favorable prognosis. In Raynaud's disease, all the fingers are affected except for the thumb. Some small necrosis (lifeless areas) can occur during an attack, leaving what are known as "rat-bite scars." After the attack, the fingers turn intensely red and swell painfully. The returning stream of blood and vitality show how painfully life and its energy can be experienced.

Symbolically, the symptoms of low blood pressure are emphasized which also mainly affects women. With the skin dying, the border to the outside world actually breaks up. At the same time, the rat-bite scars symbolize vulnerability and lack of protection in the patient's territory. She apparently cannot protect her skin. The opposite pole of openness and willingness to let something in also illustrates the vessels' extreme constriction. Such a hand is certainly anything but loving. Lynch graphically describes how hate that is primarily unconscious leads to this symptom. The ice-cold hand symbolizes the cold hatred that, when emotionally repulsed, develops within the body. The numbly stiff, dead, hands also symbolize stagnation and the inability to act. Such hands cannot make any form of contact, let alone get a grip on one's life. The learning tasks revealed in the symptoms correspond to those described in the chapter on hypotension. The problem of the skin boundaries and of acting efficiently are merely emphasized in this case.

Further Problems in the Course of the Circle

The most serious circulatory disorders are related to smoking. The most common form was discussed in the section on intermittent claudication, the intermittent laming. Gangrene has an even more drastic effect because the leg actually decays on the living body. Smoking and cardiovascular problems frequently go hand in hand because they are both symptoms of the same basic pattern, an unconscious disturbance regarding contact and enjoyment.

Part 3

I.
Cardiovascular Therapies

1.

Fundamental Considerations of Medication

The essential steps of therapy are to perceive the underlying pattern, accept it, and take the learning steps that the symptoms demand. These three steps can be supported by the various measures described in the following sections.

Apart from this approach, which admittedly requires one to have much courage and honesty with oneself as well as a sense of responsibility and strength, an abundance of orthodox and naturopathic therapies are available. These must be put to use in acute or advanced states of a disease. However, such methods cannot truly heal because that requires inner cooperation and development. Not even the most orthodox scientist would claim to be able to create well-being through the use of drugs.

The main therapeutic agent of orthodox medicine in the case of cardiac insufficiency is digitalis, which is foxglove, making it a distinctly natural remedy. This illustrates how illogical it is to make a sharp distinction between orthodox and natural medicine. For example, orthodox medicine uses cortisone, a natural hormone, as well as penicillin, which originates from the mold Aspergillus penicillium. On the other hand, many people consider homeopathy to be part of naturopathy, although the potencies[22] do not and cannot exist in nature. Homeopathy is essentially an artificial therapy—an art, at least to a certain extent.

The most important naturopathic remedies for cardiac insufficiency are crataegus (hawthorn) and convallaria (lily of the valley). Just like foxglove, these are plants whose extracts strengthen the heart. This means that no major differences exist between the orthodox and natural medicine. The later involves purely empirical medicine, even if orthodox medicine can scientifically prove its validity. In addition, the intention behind the administration of these remedies is almost identical—to eliminate the symptoms as quickly as possible and without too much difficulty.

Even if they constantly feud with each other, these two schools of medicine are very close in philosophy. The biggest difference lies between them and the medical approach presented in this book, which does not want to fight the symptoms but rather be an ally of the patient on the evolutionary path. At the moment, none of the predominant schools of medicine follows this approach. Only the concept of homeopathy is related to it. The ancient medicine of the priest-doctors, with its roots in ritual, was also based on this point of view. The same can be said for medical approaches derived from religion and esoterics.

Even though the approach presented here differs from that of orthodox medicine and naturopathy, there is no reason for them to work against each other. On the contrary, the ideas outlined in this book show how valuable scientific results can be for the interpretation of symptoms. For treatment, it is often necessary to take advice from both sides. In the case of acute heart fibrillation, however, the interpretation of the symptoms is superfluous and orthodox medicine alone has a say. For a heart that has lost its strength at the end of a strenuous life, the choice "interpret or digitalize" does not make sense. The two approaches are not mutually exclusive and do not obstruct one another. Interpretation without accompanying medical treatment is irresponsible, and drugs alone represent no more than symptomatic relief. Each of these approaches has its right time and place, and common sense determines when and how they should be applied. In addition, common sense can ease the relationship between medicine and naturopathy and create an awareness of their fundamentally different approaches to interpretive medicine. To grow through the symptoms and, in the process, make them superfluous is certainly the path with the wider perspective. However, the path of the counterpole often cannot be overlooked in the short term. In order to gather experience, in and through the body, it is ultimately important to take good care of it.

The second largest group of drugs that orthodox medicine administers for symptoms with a "nervous component" consists of psychopharmacological drugs and beta blockers. These must be viewed in a much more critical light since their overriding intention is to suppress problems and betray patients about their existence. Apart from extreme situations, such as an acute heart attack or other crises, this type of chemical tranquilization is questionable at best. It pushes true solutions further into the background. The dependency that often arises with continued use reveals the true character of this "therapy," which solves nothing and makes the patient dependent instead of free.

The action of drugs such as Valium or Librium, which are intended to have the same effect on patients, creates a "psych vegetative" decoupling. In this case, the connection between the soul and the autonomic nervous system is severed to detach the body from emotional stress. Ultimately, this may even intensify the problem, particularly for hypertensive and coronary patients who already suffer from being disconnected from their emotions. Since feelings for oneself and other people are of vital significance, chemical blocks only accentuate pharmacological loneliness. This type of treatment represents a childish approach, much like turning off the television to stop the terrible pictures of war on the news. The war itself can hardly be influenced by such an action. Chemical attempts to decouple emotions are equally ineffective, and offer no prospects for the future. To a certain extent, this also applies to natural sedatives, although these at least have the advantage of few side effects. Chemical dampers

Fundamental Considerations of Medication

merely rob the person of his stage, but the drama continues unwatched. In this respect, tranquilizers are true dampers for the healing attempts of the organism.

The most obvious alternative would be emotional relaxation. However, this requires effort and taking responsibility, which makes it less popular than other options. This method does not disconnect the soul from the body, or emotions from consciousness, which would be difficult for hypertensive and heart attack patients. Instead, contact is intensified in a healing sense. Emotions are not dampened; rather, they become more conscious and accessible so they can be worked on more efficiently. Of course, specific medical therapies (especially those for rhythmic disorders and high blood pressure) often cannot be circumvented in an acute crisis. However in the long term, patients should be aware that these drugs can only suppress symptoms. This is most obvious in the case of antiarrhythmic drugs that function anesthetically. Even if they can save lives in acute cases, they are not effective at healing.

2.

Diet

For hypertensive patients, treatment with saluretic drugs is sometimes prescribed. These are chemical substances that promote the excretion of sodium in the urine. Since salt binds with water to a considerable degree, it is disruptive in hypertension. The question of what causes the high intake of salt in most industrial societies arises. From a medical perspective, it is clear that this cannot be considered the "salt of life." It is probably the salt we are metaphorically missing, a deficiency we try to compensate for with table salt. Could it be that the soup of life has become so insipid and boring that it constantly needs salt added?

Since an excess of salt is particularly dangerous for hypertensives, its consumption must be reduced in various ways. The most simple, the salt-free diet, does not work well in practice because too many foods, such as bread, sausage, and cheese contain an abundance of salt. There would be little left for hypertensives to eat. They would need a very high level of awareness of their disorder and even greater knowledge about diet. However, if they had all these things, they probably would not be hypertensive. For this reason, even restrictions such as potato or rice diets (both are diuretic and, thus, relieve the heart and circulation) have proven more successful than attempts to eliminate salt. With respect to diet and nutritional therapies, it can be

Diet

said that the best diet is to eat nothing for a certain time, to fast, because this approach also affects the soul.

This, however, touches a central problem with all effective functional therapies. Although their intention is correct, and illuminating on a superficial level, they do not make enough allowance for deeper problems. This is especially clear in the case of obesity, which is a considerable risk factor in cardiovascular disorders. The excess weight must be reduced immediately, as books on this topic succinctly indicate. The patient simply would have to eat less. But this is precisely what he cannot do. If he were capable of doing so, he would not have fattened himself in the first place. All the risk factors are related to the pattern itself and must be entirely eliminated. Otherwise, the famous-infamous shifting of symptoms will occur within the same pattern. At the doctor's orders, one will stop smoking and instead start eating more. The two risk factors are merely exchanged and a great deal of emotional stress is added.

Salt, like nicotine and obesity, is unhealthy for both hypertensives and those with cardiac insufficiency. A relaxed life in fresh air with a healthy, natural, salt-free diet and adequate exercise and happy relationships would be best. But patients can only follow this if they discard their inner patterns and chose new ones. This type of emotional surgery may be the dream of many patients, but it is only a dream. This takes us back to the beginning of this book. In order to transform one's own pattern, several conscious steps are required: the first is to discover the pattern in one's life; the next is a willingness to accept it as the pattern one is entitled to at the moment. Only after taking these steps does it make sense to find different, more healing options for redemption. If dietary or athletic methods are applied in line with this thinking, their prospect for success is improved.

3.

Fasting as Therapy and Path

As a purely functional method, the so-called starvation diet has some major advantages compared with drugs or other diets. Such a diet has a decisive impact on the risk factors for heart attack. Nicotine abuse, high blood fats, hypertension, increased blood sugar, obesity, and lack of exercise promote a heart attack in the order listed.

During many years of attending to individuals and groups while they were fasting, 1 saw that there is no better opportunity to get a grip on nicotine consumption than during voluntary abstinence from food. Cholesterol levels and excess weight decrease with each day of a fast. According to reports from Fahmer,[23] blood fat levels are normalized after about ten days. Essential hypertension also improves rapidly, and blood pressure often returns to normal at the end of the first week. Although diabetes requires certain precautionary measures, it also improves impressively in many cases. Even a lack of exercise can easily be corrected during a fasting period because a desire for movement usually occurs. Often, the doctor supervising the fast has to make sure that the patient's enjoyment of exercise does not lead to any type of excess.

Perhaps the greatest danger involved in fasting is that type A hypertensives tend to overdo it because of their ambition.

Fasting as Therapy and Path

Although fasting is an ancient religious exercise that has been used in all ages and by all peoples, it should be considered a therapeutic measure in the case of cardiovascular disorders. As such, it requires certain rules and precautions. A doctor familiar with fasting should be consulted to supervise the fast, although it is not necessary to stay at a spa or clinic. A group situation offers major advantages, but also some disadvantages.

However, the physiological effects are only of secondary importance in the wonderful opportunity presented by fasting. The primary opportunity is the expansion of consciousness, which naturally follows. Fasting has been an important practice in all religions for good reason. Even people who begin to fast solely for medical reasons often experience inner changes and reorientation. Fasting takes one back to the center—the individual organs, as well as the whole person. Zimmerman has proven with impressive x-rays that typical "stretched-out" hearts return to their original form. Not only the heart finds its way back to the center; blood pressure also returns to its accustomed levels. Although this may be less surprising for high blood pressure than for hypotension, even low blood pressure often increases. However, it does so only after the fasting period ends, and only to the degree that the patient has faced himself.

Fasting is an ideal opportunity to take such inner steps. Carried out consciously, it includes a gentle psychotherapy that affects the body, soul, and mind equally. In order for this to happen, it is important to create the appropriate atmosphere to promote inner growth and to permit a turn toward the inner self Spas are not always the best place for this, particularly if they are populated by overweight patients who have only two themes in life: eating and losing weight.

If the inner attitude is correct, the medical advantages of fasting have an even greater effect. In addition to relieving pressure and preventing heart attack, its soothing effects include improvement of circulatory disorders and certain arrhythmias. Even an increase in the heart's strength, similar to the effect achieved with digitalis, has been observed by Fahmer when cardiac insufficiency is based on hypertension, obesity, or stress. As for the body, reduced use of the digestive system is easy on the heart. Decreased basal metabolism relieves the heart and circulation. This impressive regenerative effect is a cure for body and soul alike.

Such relaxation should be convincing to patients who are strained, exhausted, tense, or overwrought. This tendency can be promoted by further therapeutic measures. Simple exercise and relaxation methods, such as autogenous training, provide good support. There is hardly a better time than during a fast to take the first step toward meditation and other spiritual practices. Because this is a good time to start on new paths, it is also easier to leave old ones behind. Old habits and addictions are often given up incidentally during a fast. If the fast is successful, the chances are good for maintaining all aspects of the new freedom.

In this process, everything depends on the level of consciousness. A starvation diet in a clinic, carried out as a purely functional measure to fight the risk factors, will not achieve anything beyond the attempt to cut out salt. After an initial improvement, everything will return to the old patterns, and the heart will continue to suffer. Consciousness is the key to any success. In comparison with diets and other prescribed methods, fasting has the advantage of promoting the process of becoming conscious. This can lead to the beginning of taking responsibility for oneself and starting on the path to emotional development.

4.

Inner and Outer Movement

Lack of exercise is one of the risk factors that lead to heart attacks. In addition, exercise is considered the classical therapy for low blood pressure and weak circulation. In the proceeding chapters, it was explained that inner movement is the issue behind various health problems. External exercise is better than none at all, although it can only help as long as the patient actively participates in it. On the other hand, if awareness of the learning task leads to inner steps, the effect is a more reliable and lasting. The more intense this awareness is, and the better its symbolic character is understood, the more effective outer movement will be. In this respect, half an hour spent on a home trainer while thinking of something else or watching television is useless. A conscious run in the woods or even a walk brings much more "into motion."

Most appropriate, of course, is movement or exercise that consciously connects the inner and outer worlds in a ritualistic way. One example of such an exercise ritual is Tai-Chi. With its flowing movements, it is primarily focused on an awareness of one's center. Although Tai-Chi is one of the original forms of Asiatic martial arts, the movement serves as an end in itself. Today, Tai-Chi classes are offered at many centers. For the cardiac patient who has lost access to his center, this is an ideal exercise to symbolically work through his themes. Moreover, the slow, flowing movements are a good protection against exaggeration. Ambition and hectic rushing quickly become apparent and can be transformed into a harmonious flow during the circling of one's center. Tai-Chi offers an opportunity for patients with heart attack or regurgitation problems to slowly get back in shape. The goal is not to perfectly execute a complex movement, but to perform simple and conscious movements. Since, like fasting, Tai-Chi moves one toward the center, these two therapies are effective in combination. While one practices the outer exercise, his inner life also takes on a new shape.

An even simpler symbolic exercise, which also focuses exclusively on the center, is the painting of mandalas. Mandalas are circular forms that exist in all cultures and are still used for meditation in the East. In the West, they are somewhat lifeless remnants of a lost tradition, as for example in the rosette windows of Gothic cathedrals. While the physical demands of Tai-Chi are minor, painting a mandala requires nothing except the conscious holding of a colored pencil. Precisely because it is so simple and childlike, this exercise can have a tremendous effect. However, one must inwardly outrun his shadow and open up to the process. Constantly focusing on symbols of the center animates one's heart in a mysterious way and can put people into motion who have been stagnant for a long time.

5.

Spiritual-Emotional Exercises on the Path to the Healed Heart

With Anahata, the heart chakra, the heart was always at the center of spiritual exercises. The heart prayer of the Eastern Orthodox Church, which repeats the name of the Redeemer like a mantra in the heart, is one example. A modern variation of this prayer or meditation can be found in the book on heart meditations by Siegfried Scharf.[24]

Ultimately, the best exercise is simply to listen to one's own heart. This is exactly what all heart symptoms suggest, and sometimes even force upon one. However, in the present era, the simplest things have become the most difficult. Or, perhaps, they have always been difficult, if one considers Goethe's words: "Humans cannot forgive the truth for being so simple." So it may be worthwhile to use outside aids.

*Medi*tation aims for the middle, just as *medi*cine originally did. There is only one center, but many techniques and exercises exist for approaching it. The heart patient's problem is his loss of center and, with it, loss of purpose in life. In this respect, meditation can become the central re*medy* or *medi*cine for him since it leads on the path to this center, to the heart.

The Benedictine monk and philosopher Steindl-Rast[25] called the heart the organ to find meaning. He recommended that one listen with the heart and attune it to the call of Creation. In Steindl-Rast's opinion, when this listening stops taking place, and thus a person can no longer obey God, life becomes absurd (Latin *absurdus* means absolutely deaf). Deafness that affects the emotions, and thereby one's interactions with the surrounding world, is characteristic of many heart patients, especially type A patients. These patients are deaf to the language of their hearts and lack the ability to fantasize and express emotions. Under the term *alexithymia*. Professor Lynch has compiled the special characteristics of these patients and expressed their characteristics in words similar to those of Steindl-Rast: "They have no words to describe what they do not feel." For Lynch, as well, sense and sensuousness are closely related. What is non-sensuous can quickly turn into nonsense. The path of the heart and meditation cannot be regarded simply as functional methods, like swallowing a pill three times as day. First, however, one must recognize that something is missing deep within the heart.

The term *meditation* has an Eastern ring to it. The East has actually kept it alive in its relatively healthy traditions. Yet, its roots can be found equally in the Western cultures. One just has to dig a bit in order to find it there. However, because it seems easier to adopt Eastern forms of meditation—which are offered everywhere today—many people have chosen this path. Nevertheless, if a patient begins to meditate because of his symptoms, it may be easier to adopt a Western form of meditation, especially one that can be found in the old mystery cults. It is likely that the medicine of classical antiquity was also familiar with this form of guided meditation. Those seeking healing would go to a place such as the Aesculapian temple, where they would be prepared and put in the right frame of mind. Purification rituals and spiritual exercises mainly took place in the inner world of imagination and imagery. The high priest lead the soul on the path of healing by guiding him through the inner world of archetypes. During the decisive ritual, the healing sleep, the seeker spent one night sleeping in a special place in the temple. Prepared on the inner level and guided into the realm of inner images, he was able to dream the solution to his problem.

The extraordinary success of this ancient form of medicine was based on the fact that it penetrated to the root of the symptom, creating insights and providing inspiration. The process was aided by the intimate access people of that era had to their inner realms. They were considerably more open to the shadow of human existence than we are today. In their theater—and it is no coincidence that the Greek word *theos,* meaning God, is hidden in this word—tragedies predominated. The basic theme of the plays was the guilt of humanity. In contrast, today people prefer comedies. They do not want to deal with the shadow side of life in general, let alone their own shadows. This is why they are both unwilling and unprepared to experience this aspect, and instead project it in the form of external enemies and inner symptoms.

In many respects, current psychotherapies attempt to duplicate the path of ancient initiation rituals by assisting those who seek healing to find access to the deep layers of their soul. Guided meditations and mind travel play a major role in this process. For the cardiac patient, they also fulfill the important task of helping him find access to his fantasies and feelings once again. In an age characterized by a mechanistic view of the world, with strictly causal thinking, this is no easy venture. Yet, it is often the only way. For this reason, psychotherapy may be the best path for a symptom that appears first on a purely physical level. However, it must be a form of psychotherapy that builds on analogous thinking and access to inner images. The inner dialog, which lakes place in the heart and the vessels, must be transformed into a language the patient can understand and speak. Although this may sound like learning a foreign language, it is only a matter of, once again, learning one's mother tongue—the language of the heart. If a person is not conscious of his feelings, he cannot convey them to others. This means that he is unable to communicate. He must first learn to express what is bothering him and, at the same time, remain conscious of his body. Gently relaxed breathing is a good approach to this goal.

The psychotherapist faces a difficult task that puts into question her usual role. If she remains in the usual position of authority, she will tend to intensify the problems of the type-A patient. As long as the therapist demands to be superior, she will not be able to listen because she must constantly prepare for battle with such patients. On the other hand, if the therapist is willing to find a balance of authority by revealing her own vulnerability and placing herself on the same level as the patient, true communication can occur. Only then does the patient have a chance to once again find a home within his own physical house. With no contact to his heart and feelings, he lives in a form of inner exile. While serious cardiovascular problems may require psychotherapy as the first step on the path of the heart, one can often start out on this path by oneself. For the true answers can only be found in one's own heart.

II.
The Path of the Heart

1.

Love

Completely independent of the physical condition of the heart, it is never too late to take the path of the heart. Even if one has taken far-reaching detours and lost sight of the central goal, it is not too late. Through the mouth of Ezekiel, the biblical God pardons His people who have greatly distanced themselves: "A new heart I will give you and a new spirit I will put within you." (Ez. 36.26)

The heart, as the center and place of love, always awaits. When it draws attention to itself with physical or emotional symptoms, this is merely a sign that it is longingly waiting for its owners' return. The path it wants to show us is the path of love, which leads through thick and thin from the opposites of the polar world to the unity of Paradise. The heart is the gateway to this dimension which is inconceivable to us and is known, in different cultures, as the Self, Nirvana, the Tao, Kether, Brahman, Allah, the Kingdom of Heaven, Paradise, or Unity—all many names for the indescribable One.

Of Love
Then, said Almitra, Speak to us of Love.
And he raised his head and looked upon the people,
and there fell a stillness upon them.
And with a great voice he said:

Love

When love beckons to you follow him, Though his ways are hard and steep.
And when his wings enfold you, yield to him, Though his pinions may wound you.
And when he speaks to you, believe in him, Though his voice may shatter your dreams as the north wind, lays waste the garden.
For even as love crowns you, so shall he crucify you.
Even as he is for your growth, so is he for your pruning.
Even as he ascends to your height and caresses your tenderest branches that quiver in the sun,
So shall he descend to your roots and shake them in their clinging to the earth.
Like sheaves of com, he gathers you into himself.
He threshes you to make you naked.
He sifts you to free you from your husks.
He grinds you to whiteness.
He kneads you until you are pliant;
And then he assigns you to his sacred fire, that you may become sacred bread for God's sacred feast.
All these things shall love do unto you that you may know the secrets of your heart, and in that knowledge become a fragment of Life's heart.
But if in your fear you would seek only love's peace and love's pleasure,
Then it is better for you that you cover your nakedness and pass out of love's threshing-floor.
Into the seasonless world where you shall laugh, but not all of your laughter, and weep, but not all of your tears.
Love gives naught but itself and takes naught but from itself

Heart-Aches

> Love possesses not nor would it be possessed;
> For love is sufficient unto love.
> When you love you should not say, "God is in my heart, " but rather, "I am in the heart of God. "

—K. Gibran, *The Prophet.*

Endnotes

1. In his honor, even doctors today abbreviate the blood pressure with RR. RR 120/80 therefore represents a normal blood pressure with an upper value of 120 and a lower value of 80. The meaning of this will be explained in the section on the circulatory system.
2. This becomes even more clear in the definition of health by WHO, whereby health is a state free of physical, mental, and social suffering.
3. A more extensive explanation of the idea of polarity and the topic of good and evil can be found in Dethlefsen, T. & Dahlke, R., *Krankheit als Weg,* Bertelsmann: Munich, 1986.
4. Christ addressed the Devil as the Lord of this World as he left his disciples after the Last Supper.
5. With this, the two basic principles are searched—the sunlike principle of the heart and the venus-like principle of the kidneys.
6. The name refers to the Papal mitra, which the valve with its two cusps resembles. In comparison, its counterpart in the right heart has three cusps and is called the tricuspid.
7. Condrau, G., & Gassmann, M., *Das verletzte Herz.* Zurich 1989.
8. Lynch, J.J., *The Body Response to Human Dialogue,* Basic Books: New York, 1985.
9. A detailed treatment of this topic is found in Dethlefsen, T. & Dahlke, R., *Krankheit als Weg,* Bertelsmann: Munich, 1986.
10. Much could be said about allergies. But since they have already been discussed in *Krankheit als Weg* (see above). I would just like to comment on a few special characteristics necessary for the better understanding of the topic.

11 Stevenson, I., *20 Cases Suggestive of Reincarnation,* Univ. Press of Va: Charlottesville, 1980.

12 A detailed introduction to this way of thinking and the corresponding world view is found in the books Dethlefsen, T., *Healing Power of Illness. The Meaning of Symptoms & How to Interpret Them,* Shaftesbury: Element, 1990 and Dethlefsen, T. & Dahlke, R., *Krankheit als Weg,* Bertelsmann: Munich, 1986. Even the statements made by these two titles show that this is a matter of opportunities and paths instead of something like the assignment of blame.

13 Kübler-Ross, E., *On Children and Death,* S&S Trade, 1993.

14 Kyber, M., *Die drei Lichter der kleinen Veronica,* Heyne: Munich. 1984.

15 In recent years, new, less rigid valves which no longer require blood liquefaction for the remainder of a patient's life have become available for some patients.

16 Catecholamine is a term for certain amines such as adrenaline, noradrenaline, and dopamine.

17 Klepzig, H., *Herz~ and Fefäßkrankheiten,* Thieme: Stuttgart, 1972.

18 Richter, H.-E. & Beckmann, D., *Herzneurose,* Thieme: Stuttgart, 1969.

19 Lynch, J.J., *The Body's Response to Human Dialogue,* Basic Books: New York, 1985.

20 Condrau, G., & Gassmann, M., *Das verletzte Herz,* Zurich 1989.

21 Alexander, F., *Psychosomatische Medizin,* DeGruyter: Berlin, 1985.

22 For homeopathic medications potencies are created through a certain method of diluting and shaking the remedy.

23 Fahmer, H., *Fasten als Therapie,* Stuttgart 1985.

24 Scharf, S., *Die Praxis der Herzensmeditation,* Aurum: Freiburg, 1983.
25 Steindl-Rast, D., *A Listening Heart. A Art of Co?ntemplative Living,* Crossroad: New York, 1983.

Bibliography

Alexander, F., *Medical Value of Psychoanalysis*, Inti. Univ. Pr: Chicago, 1985.
Alexander, F., *Psychosomatische Medizin*, DeGruyter: Berlin, 1985.
Al Huang, C., *Beginning TaiJi*, Celestial Arts: Milbrae,CA, 1989.
Brautigam, W., & Christians, P.: *Topics of Psychosomatic Research*, S. Karger: Basel, 1973.
Condrau, G., & Gassmann, M., *Das verletzte Herz*, Zurich 1989.
Dahlke, R., *Gewichtsprobleme*, Knaur-Tb.: Munich, 1989.
—, *Der Mensch und die Welt sind eins*, Knaur: Munich 1987
—, *Bewußt fasten*, Goldmann: Munich, 1996.
—, *Verdauungsprobleme*, Knaur-Tb.: Munich, 1990.
R. Dahlke & K. Von Martius, *Mandalas of the World*, Sterling: New York, 1992.
Dahlke, R. & M., *Die Psychologic des blauen Dunstes*, Knaur-Tb.: Munich, 1989.
Dethlefsen, T., *Healing Power of Illness. The Meaning of Symptoms S. How to Interpret Them*, Shaftesbury: Element, 1990.
Dethlefsen, T. & Dahlke, R., *Krankheit als Weg*, Bertelsmann: Munich, 1986.
Fahmer, H., *Fasten als Therapie*, Stuttgart 1985.
Gibran, K., *The Prophet*, Knopf: New York, 1926
Klein, N. & Dahlke, R., *Das senkrechte Weltbild.Symbolisches Denken in astrologischen Urprinzipien*, Hugendubel: Munich, 1988.
Klepzig, H., *Herz- und Gefäßkrankheiten*, Thieme: Stuttgart, 1972.
Kübler-Ross, E., *On Children and Death*, S&S Trade, 1993
Kyber, M., *Die drei Lichter der kleinen Veronica*, Heyne: Munich, 1984.
Lynch, J.J., *The Body's Response to Human Dialogue*, Basic Books: New York, 1985.
Richter, H.-E. & Beckmann, D., *Herzneurose*, Thieme: Stuttgart, 1969.
Scharf, S., *Die Praxis der Herzensmeditation*, Aurum: Freiburg, 1983.

Steindl-Rast, D.,*A Listening Heart. A Art of Comtemplative Living,* Crossroad: New York, 1983.

Stevenson, I., *20 Cases Suggestive of Reincarnation,* Univ. Press of Va: Charlottesville, 1980.

Index

A

Acetylcholine 174, 228
Adams-Stokes seizures 189
Adrenal gland 112
Adrenaline 112, 170, 182, 228, 257
Adventitia 225
AIDS 5
Albigenses 17
Alexander, Franz 105, 271
Alexithymia 300
Allergic reaction 122-124, 154
American Heart Association 6
Amniotic fluid 141
Anahata 15, 56, 220, 299
Anastomoses 246
Anesthetization 187
Aneurysm 101
Angina pector 170
Anima 91, 255. See also Animus
Animus 255. See also Anima
Antibiotics 120
Anticoagulants 114, 158
Antigens 122-126, 131, 167
Antispasmodic remedies 114
Anxiety neurotic 11
Aorta 74, 141, 146-150, 156, 158, 165-166, 283
Aortic regurgitation 147, 165, 167
Aortic stenosis 155
Archetypes 94, 301
Aristotle 15
Armor heart 126, 129
Arrhythmia 108, 111, 174-175, 178, 182, 184-185, 190, 194
Arterial calcification 88
Arteriosclerosis 5-6, 88, 142, 146, 194, 260, 262
Arthritic pain 126
Artificial respiration 188
Artificial valve 158
Aspirin 158
Athletic heart 82-83
Atrial fibrillation 184
Atrial flutter 126, 184-185
Atrioventricular block 194
Atrioventricular node 77, 171-172, 188
Atrioventricular valve 125
Atrium 73-75, 79, 125, 141, 151, 159, 165, 167, 171, 180, 182, 184-186, 188
Autogenous training 169, 296
AV node 77

B

Balloon catheters 19
Baroreceptors 227
Bible 15-17, 20, 38, 39, 40-42, 54, 65-66, 164, 189
Biofeedback 169
Blood 6-11, 14-5, 18-19, 48, 50-51, 56-58, 71, 73-76, 79-81, 84-86, 88-89, 98-102, 104-105, 108, 110-114, 126-127, 133, 141-142, 146-148, 150-168, 174, 181, 184, 186-190, 194-196, 198, 202-203, 205, 212, 225-239, 243-284, 291-295, 295, 297, 312-313
Blood cells 56, 126, 158
Blood clot 89, 247
Blood congestion 244
Blood liquefaction 158, 186, 313
Blood pressure 6-9, 15, 18-19, 51, 79, 80, 81, 84-85, 88, 98-101, 105, 114, 148, 155, 166, 168, 174, 194-196, 212, 225-228, 231, 233, 238, 248, 250, 251, 254-264-297, 312. See also Hypertension, Hypotension
Blood sugar 294
Bradyarrhythmia 174
Brahmaputra 15
Brautigam 209, 307
Broken heart 107
Brown atrophy 202
Buddha 34, 253
Buddhism 230
Bypass 19, 92

C

Caffeine 182
Cancer 5
Capillaries 166, 225-226
Cardiac arrest 187, 197, 218
Cardiac arrhythmia 174, 175, 178, 182
Cardiac defect 75
Cardiac enlargement 81-85

Index

Cardiac infarction 108. See also Heart attack
Cardiac inflammation 128
Cardiac insufficiency 190, 194, 288, 289, 293, 295. See also Insufficiency
Cardiac neurosis 208-220
Cardiac output 189, 227-228
Cardiac plexus 79
Cardiac septum 75
Cardiophobia 209
Cardiopulmonary system 73
Carotid artery 147-148, 166
Catecholamines 174
Cathari 17, 55
Catholicism 231
Catholics 16
Chakra 15, 56, 220, 299
Chemoreceptors 227
Cholesterol 88, 114
Christ 34, 39, 41, 51, 55, 65-66, 140, 231, 312
Christian church 17, 58
Chronic emaciation 202
Chronic infections 143
Church fathers 140
Cicero 44
Circulatory collapse 111, 112
Circulatory shock 111
Circulatory System 14, 102, 223
Coarctation 147-150, 283
Cold feet 30, 59, 95, 148, 237
Condrau 104, 271, 307, 312, 313
Congenital heart defects 150
Congenital symptoms 139
Congested heart 153
Congestive catarrh 196
Congestive heart failure 194, 196
Congestive pneumonia 196
Constriction 10, 19, 73, 86-91, 94-95, 105, 109, 127, 147-152, 160, 165, 190, 195, 210, 237, 260, 272-273, 277, 284
Convallaria 289
Cor bovinum 165
Coronary arteriosclerosis 194
Coronary sclerosis 7-8, 88-89, 102, 182, 260
Coronary vessels 7, 19, 71, 73, 87-91, 95, 102, 105, 109, 113, 166, 190
Cortisone 134-137, 183, 288
Cramps 243, 244
Craniosacral 227

Crataegus 289
Crescendo murmurs 151
Cupid 45
Cusp valves 131
Cyanosis 152, 159, 194, 203

D

Death 5, 7, 13-15, 51, 53, 64, 71, 75, 90, 94, 97-98, 100-103, 107, 111, 113, 116-117, 120, 127-130, 171, 187-188, 192, 197, 199, 201, 211-212, 215, 218, 227
Defibrillation 186-187
Depression 53
Diastole 73, 76
Diet 292-294, 296
Digitalis 182-183, 288, 295
Digiti mortui 284
Dilation 195
Dizziness 152, 180, 181, 185, 233, 237
Dostoyevski 44
Dreams 31-32, 181, 244, 305
Ductus arteriosus 141, 146, 147
Dystrophy 202

E

Eastern medicine 79
Eastern Orthodox Church 16, 299
Eastern traditions 56, 139
ECG. See Electrocardiogram
Eckehart 44
Edema 244
Egyptians 15
Electrocardiogram 19, 76
Electroshock 111
Embolism 89, 101, 127, 158, 186, 245, 247
Endocarditis 122, 126-127, 131, 155
Endocarditis lenta 131
Energy centers. See Chakra
Enlargement of the heart 125, 165, 190
Epilepsy 185, 189
Erysipelas 122
Esoteric psychology 29
Essential hypertension 294
Estrogen 89
Exercise 89, 104, 114, 175, 176, 226, 249, 275, 293-299
Extrasystoles 130, 131, 182-186, 210

F

Fasting 294-296, 298
Fatty degeneration 203-204
Faust 35-36
Feminist movement 255
Fibrillation 47, 100, 108, 111-112, 126, 128, 151, 182, 184-188, 194, 197, 289
Fibrosis 202
Flutter 99, 126, 128, 182-187, 194
Fontane, Theodor 43
Foxglove 288-289
Freud 209
Friedmann 105

G

Galloping heart 176, 218
Galloping rhythm 47, 98
Gilgamesh 15
Glomerulonephritis 122
Gnostics 17
Goethe 35, 43, 52, 299
Grail 164, 213, 231
Greeks 15
Groddeck, Georg 20

H

Hairy heart 126, 129
Harvey, William 18-19, 72
Heart attack 5, 25, 49, 73, 86, 88, 90, 97-117, 128, 131, 156, 166, 182, 186, 211, 213, 260, 263, 272, 290-298
Heart block 188-190
Heart catheterization 187
Heart defect 127, 141, 144, 146, 150, 155, 160, 165
Heart failure 51, 82, 84, 97, 99, 179, 187, 188, 194, 196-198
Heart frequency 170
Heart Inflammation 122. See also Inflammation
Heart Prayer 16
Heart racing 48, 181
Heart rate 173, 174, 178
Heart regurgitation 126
Heart rhythm 184
Heart sac 50, 100, 126, 136
Heart septum 57, 141
Heart surgery 142, 187
Heart transplantation 200

Heart valves 163
Hectic heart 108
Heine, Heinrich 44, 48
Hemalysis 158
High blood pressure. See Hypertension
Hildegard of Bingen 43
Horst Rüdiger 50
Hyperalgesia 210
Hypertension 168, 190, 256-263, 271, 273, 283, 284, 292, 294, 296
Hypertrophic muscles 83
Hypochondriasis 213-215
Hypotension 243, 250, 253, 254, 257, 259, 284, 295
Hysterical heart 210

I

Idiopathic 131
Immunosuppressives 200
Inflammation 120-138, 244-246, 283
Insufficiency 190, 194, 199, 203, 243, 288, 289, 293, 296
Insufficiency at rest 194, 199
Intermittent claudication 260, 285
Intima 264

J

Jesus 16
Jung, C.G. 31, 255

K

Kidney inflammation 122
Klepzig, H. 184, 187, 249, 307, 313
Korotkow 18
Kübler-Ross, Elizabeth 144, 307, 313
Kulenkampff 209
Kyber, Manfred 307

L

Lack of sleep 182
Lactate dehydrogenase 111
Language of symptoms 32
Latent infections 122
Librium 290
Lipids 88, 104
Liquefaction 111, 158, 186, 313
Locus minoris resistentiae 122

Index

Loss of consciousness 185, 186, 189
Love 3, 10-17, 39, 40, 44-67, 78, 81, 84, 95, 96, 107, 118, 119, 159, 178, 186, 203, 212, 213, 220, 253, 265, 267, 272, 274, 275, 304, 305, 306
Low blood pressure 84, 148, 233, 238, 248, 251, 254, 255, 257, 280, 282, 284, 295, 297. See also Hypotension
Luther, Martin 42
Lynch, J.J. 107, 264, 266, 267, 268, 270, 275, 277, 284, 300, 307, 312, 313

M

May, Rollo 10
Meditation 30, 173, 277, 296, 298, 299, 300
Mephistopheles 35
Mitral regurgitation 125, 165, 196
Mitral stenosis 151, 155
Mitral valve 74, 165
Morphine 111, 113, 114, 135, 136
Myocardial contractions 195
Myocardial infarction 49
Myocardial rupture 100
Myocarditis 122, 127, 130, 182, 183, 187, 190

N

Naturopathy 248, 288-290
Nervous system 78, 170, 174, 181, 195, 227, 228, 259, 260, 290
Nicotine 182, 293, 294
Nitrates 92
Nitroglycerin 19
Noradrenaline 228, 313

O

Obesity 203, 204, 293, 294, 296
Orthodox medicine 4, 22, 26, 33, 42, 51, 79, 91, 104, 111, 112, 114, 132, 134, 135, 137, 157, 176, 180, 183, 184, 186, 187, 191, 213, 214, 239, 248, 250, 288, 289, 290
Ox heart 165

P

Pacemaker 172, 191, 192, 193
Painkillers 135, 137
Paracelsus 9, 18
Paradise 23, 24, 44, 57, 58, 76, 142, 304
Paroxysmal Tachycardia vi, 180
Pascal, Blaise 43
Patent ductus arteriosus 146, 147
Pathogens 26, 120, 121, 122, 123, 130, 131, 132, 135, 230, 245
Pendulum 229
Penicillin 132, 288
Pericarditis 122, 126, 128, 129, 131, 136
Pheochromocytoma 283
Physics 26, 27, 28, 29, 63, 264, 267
Pickwickian syndrome 203
Pius XI 16
Plaque 88, 89
Polycythemia 152
Polyglobulism 195
Postcommissurotomy syndrome 154
Precapillary sphincters 226
Pressoreceptors 227
Prosthesis 157, 158
Psychology iv, 26, 29, 31
Psychotherapy 24, 30, 143, 200, 209, 270, 295, 301, 302
Pulmonary alveoli 102
Pulmonary circulation 142, 146, 168
Pulmonary congestion 142, 165, 195
Pulmonary edema 102, 152, 155, 196, 198
Pulmonary embolism 247
Pulmonary regurgitation 168
Pulmonary stenosis 160
Purkinje's fibers 172

R

Racing heart 49, 128, 176, 177, 178, 180, 181, 186, 212
Radionics 229
Raynaud's disease 284
Regurgitation 125, 126, 127, 147, 148, 152, 155, 164, 165, 167, 168, 196, 298
Reimann 209
Reincarnation 308, 313
Rheumatic Carditis vi, 122

Rheumatic fever 122, 124, 125, 126, 139, 159, 165, 167
Rhythmic disorders 192, 291
Richter, H.E. 210, 211, 307, 313
Right atrium 74, 79, 159, 167
Right ventricle 74, 142, 146, 159, 167, 203
Rigor mortis 13
Ringeis 18
Riva-Rocci 18
Roemheld's syndrome 205
Rosenmann 105

S

Sacred Heart of Jesus 16
Saint-Exupery 46
Saint Francis of Assisi 251
Salt 7, 104, 114, 292, 293, 296
Saluretic drugs 292
Satan 65, 66
Scarlet fever 122
Scharf, Siegfried 299
Schiller, Friedrich von 43
Schopenhauer, Arthur 44
Sclerosis 88
Septal defect 141
Septum 57, 75, 76, 141, 142, 146, 147. See also Cardiac Septum
Sexuality 59, 148, 238
Shadow 25, 26, 30, 31, 32, 36, 57, 58, 66, 67, 82, 85, 89, 121, 213, 217, 234, 239, 243, 244, 254, 255, 281, 298, 301
Shakespeare, William 48
Sinoatrial node 76, 77, 78
Solomon 17
Sore throat 122
Spasm of the coronary vessels 113
Sphincters 226, 228
Spider-burst veins 243
Sports 82
Steindl-Rast, D. 300
Steiner, Rudolf 190
Stenosis 127, 150-160, 165, 167, 168, 196
Stevenson, Ian 140
Streptococci 122, 123, 124, 125, 131
Stress 51, 104, 110, 112, 134, 142, 143, 146, 152, 155, 157, 170, 228, 257, 264, 290, 293, 296
Stroke 71, 112, 150, 179, 182, 190, 260, 284

Sympathetic nervous system 170, 174, 181, 195, 259
Symptom 4, 9-11, 22-37, 58, 82-85, 89, 93, 94, 96, 101, 115, 120, 131, 140, 144, 147, 152, 153, 159, 160, 163, 175, 184, 186, 199, 202, 205, 209, 234, 237, 238, 244, 251, 254, 256, 263, 266, 273, 282, 284, 301
Synchronicity 26
Systole 74, 76, 100

T

Tachycardia 180, 181, 210
Tai-Chi 253, 297, 298
Templars 55
Tendon fibers 126, 127, 131
Teresa of Avila 16
Thoracolumbar 227
Thrombophlebitis 245
Thrombosis 89, 101, 102, 158, 241, 245, 246, 247
Thyroid hyperactivity 176
Tissue fluid 125, 167, 168
Tolerance insufficiency 194
Tonsillitis 122
Tranquilizers 114, 176, 209, 291
Tree of Knowledge 24
Tricuspidal regurgitation 167
Tricuspidal stenosis 159
Tricuspid valve 74
Tuberculosis 5, 6
Twitching heart 49
Type A 211, 266, 294, 300

U

Ulcer 30, 244

V

Vagus 174, 180, 227, 228, 236, 259
Valium 290
Valvular defect 126, 166, 167, 196
Varicose veins 246
Vascular tree 225, 226
Vasospasms 111
Vedas 15
Vena cava 74
Ventricle 73-75, 101, 125, 141, 142, 146, 151, 154-156, 159, 165, 167, 171, 180, 182, 184, 188, 189, 194, 198, 203

Ventricular activation 188
Ventricular failure 195
Venus 45, 272

W

Western esoterics 230
WHO 6

Z

Ziegler, Alfred 13
Zimmerman 295

www.ingramcontent.com/pod-product-compliance
Lightning Source LLC
Chambersburg PA
CBHW011408070526
44586CB00021B/2575